Dale Stone's CHOOSE LIFE is an inspiring testament to the sanctity of human life from conception to the grave, written in a moving poetic style. How to feel about the sanctity of all human life is as important as what to know about it and what to do for it.
Rabbi David Novak, Vice-President, Jewish Pro-Life Foundation

CHOOSE LIFE is a powerful document recommending the preservation of life. Our Creator has placed in the DNA of every species instructions which direct it to continue living. Until the passing of Roe v. Wade it made sense in civilized society that if one human life takes another human life, the guilty should be punished. The tools and vacuums abortionists use are mostly made from metal. The Bible says *"If one strikes someone with an iron implement so that he dies, he is a murderer. The murderer should surely be put to death"* (Numbers 35:16f). ***"He who sheds blood, by man shall his blood be shed"*** (Genesis 9:6). **There is no difference in the amount of guilt if someone kills a child in the womb (abortion) or kills a child who is already born (infanticide).** Abortionists have a double standard. God forbid if pro-life literature shows photos of aborted body parts. How do abortionists react when someone described in THE TRASH MAN'S SURPRISE (p.103) smells death in a partially ripped garbage bag and opens it to reveal it is filled with aborted body parts? Abortionists could care less. Many of Dale's poems retell actual conversations he has had with those who have had an abortion experience. He documents that both hormonal based contraception and abortion are not "safe". He suggests counselors earn $600 when they guide a woman to put her child up for adoption. And a woman who gives her child up for adoption gets $2,500 paid by the person(s) who adopts her innocent child. The **L**ove **Y**our **A**mazing **M**om **P**rogram redirects 3% of the annual income tax her children paid from the IRS to her. These programs will help correct the imbalance of Americans working and being retired. CHOOSE LIFE could be an award winning movie.
Anita Kiekhaefer, Photo documentarian and teacher of Hebrew Bible literature, with most work performed in Israel.

Your message NEEDS to be read and understood. It seems that many who were raised to respect Judeo Christian values are just caving in the face of the tsunami of popular culture that has totally abandoned its foundation in Biblical truth.
Paul Strand, President Emeritus and Missionary Training Consultant for Bethany's GlobeServe

i

Children can often come at inconvenient times disrupting one's plans educationally, financially, vocationally and in many other ways. If we had let any of these things determine whether to let our pregnancies go to term, we would not have six amazing kids who have grown up to be such a positive force for good in this world: two engineers, one business owner, one airline pilot, one entrepreneur and school teacher plus their loving spouses and parents. We were way below the poverty level. I had lots of health challenges. Everything pointed to our not having children. Often our greatest challenges in life become our mission in life. This was our case and is now our greatest joy and blessing. Having volunteered in a women's clinic I saw firsthand the heartache of women who had chosen abortion over life. I appreciate Dale's heart of love and caring for others and the wisdom he shares in this book. **For those considering an abortion,** know the clinic will likely not offer to show you an ultrasound of your child or listen to his or her heartbeat. **The next book you should read is this one!** Meticulously review the questions inside the front and back covers with your abortion provider.

Marilyn Plumb, Nutrition Educator, NeoLife,
plumblinenutrition@gmail.com

———————————

What a truly informative look at abortion from all sides of the spectrum. It tugs at the heart to read poems from the expectant mother, the child and the father's viewpoints. The poem, DAD'S REGRETS (p.28) was especially touching as everything seems to be centered around the mother's regrets over time. It never occurred to me that the dad would suffer, too. I was surprised to get the view from the workers and picketers as well. A person doesn't stop to think how much it must affect them to feel so helpless. I liked how on page 62 it went into the different options in detail and later gave a list of the famous people who were adopted. For some reason that really stuck with me.

It was good to read poems about love and the poem, A FATHER'S PRAYER (p.88) again brought the dad into the picture. In a way it shows the overview of what a young girl could have if she doesn't have the abortion. She may not have it with the then father, but someday… somehow… it will happen. Also another view from a sibling in the poem, I PRAY I HAVE A LITTLE BROTHER OF MY OWN (p.90), completes a circle of what life could be if a loving mother would choose life for her baby.

The poem, MAKE LOVE YOUR CHOICE (p.230) says, **"Your lips are made to kiss your child. Your arms are made for hugs."** What a great line. It tells us that when all is said and done their baby only needs their love and not material things like the world wants us all to think.

Your book was great. I still can't get over how you got the views from all angles and you show the love from every side as well. God bless.

Sue Lueck Carlson, Poet, www.heavensrollcall.com

———————————

Choose Life!

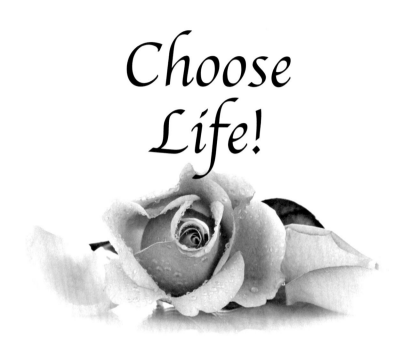

By Dale M. Stone

Cover Design by: Lakeside Press
Editor: Carol Lenhart

ABORTION (like suicide) IS A PERMANENT SOLUTION TO A TEMPORARY PROBLEM.

An unborn child isn't just a potential human being, he or she is a human baby with great potential.

"The emotional turmoil that this procedure inevitably causes the physician and staff…there is no possibility of denial of an act of destruction by the operator. The sensation of dismemberment flows through the forceps like an electric current." Hern's job was to train his colleagues how to ignore the negative emotions they felt while killing innocent babies so they could keep making money for the abortion community. (Warren Hern, MD p.167)

"O Lord my God, I take refuge in You. Save and deliver me from all who pursue me. For they will tear me like a lion. And they will rip me to pieces with no one to rescue me" (Psalm 7:1,2).

"Whoever destroys a soul, it is considered as if he destroyed an entire world. And whoever saves a life, it is considered as if he saved an entire world" (Mishnah Sanhedrin 4:9; Babylonian Talmud, Sanhedrin 37a).

"Adonai, Adonai, God, compassionate and gracious, slow to anger, abundant in kindness and truth…Who preserves kindness for a thousand generations, Who forgives iniquity, sin and error, and Who cleanses" (Exodus 34:6-7).

"What good will it be for someone to gain the whole world, yet forfeit their soul" (Matthew 16:26)?

"Never rule out a goal because you think it's unattainable. Be audacious" (Ray Dalio).

"Perseverance is the foundation of all actions" (Lao Tzu).

"The best way out is always through" (Robert Frost).

"God is our refuge and strength a very present help in trouble" (Psalm 45:1).

"We are afflicted in every way, but not crushed; perplexed, but not driven to despair; persecuted, but not forsaken; struck down, but not destroyed" (2 Corinthians 4:8).

*"This day I call the heavens and the earth as witnesses against you that I have set before you life and death, blessings and curses. **Now choose life, so that you and your children may live** and that you may love the Lord your God, listen to his voice, and hold fast to him"* (Deuteronomy 30:19-20).

"I have created him for My glory. I have formed him" (Isaiah 43:7).

On page 204 of her well researched book, 2020 THE TURNAWAY STUDY (ten years a thousand women) Diana Greene Foster, PhD asked, how long after the abortion was denied, did it take for one-third of the mothers to stop wanting an abortion? "One week after being denied an abortion, nearly two-thirds of the women reported they still wanted an abortion. But six months later, when all had given birth, just one in eight (13%) wish they could have had an abortion. Five years later, only one in twenty-five (4%) wish they could have had an abortion." (p.202)

The percentage of American women over age 45 who have had an abortion is the same for Christians as for women who don't claim to have a relationship with the Lord, i.e. "One out of three." Women and men who are considering having an abortion have it in their power to make the most loving choice and birth their unborn child. Then they can decide to keep him or her or to select adoption. Family members and true friends have it in their power to tell the mother and father experiencing a crisis pregnancy, "I will stand by you as you face this unexpected blessing."

"DO NOT WITHHOLD GOOD FROM THOSE TO WHOM IT IS DUE, WHEN IT IS IN YOUR POWER TO ACT" (Proverbs 3:27-35).

"THOU SHALT NOT KILL" (literally, commit murder) (Exodus 20:13).

"FOR I KNOW THE PLANS I HAVE FOR YOU, SAYS THE LORD, PLANS FOR WELFARE AND NOT FOR EVIL, TO GIVE YOU A FUTURE AND A HOPE." (Jeremiah 29:11).

"THERE ARE SIX THINGS THAT THE LORD HATES, SEVEN THAT ARE AN ABOMINATION TO HIM: HAUGHTY EYES, A LYING TONGUE, AND HANDS THAT SHED INNOCENT BLOOD A HEART THAT DEVISES WICKED PLANS, FEET THAT MAKE HASTE TO RUN TO EVIL, A FALSE WITNESS WHO BREATHES OUT LIES, AND ONE WHO SOWS DISCORD AMONG BROTHERS" (Proverbs 6:16-19).

Printed and bound by
Lakeside Press | Minnesota
www.lakesidecreates.com | 1-800-371-5849

Disclaimer

The information in this book is shared for educational purposes. My poems
and research are designed to direct readers away from risking the dangers
of abortion and motivate them to always CHOOSE LIFE. This book is not
written to diagnose or give medical or psychological advice or treatment.
Please bring your medical questions to a licensed physician. Make use
of the trained counselors listed in the resource section. They are eager to
hear about your challenges and to encourage you. Knowledge is power.
CHOOSE LIFE will empower you. Regretfully not all emails may be
answered, but all will be read.

Dedication

The greatest of riches aren't dollars
or stocks, buildings, silver or gold.
The greatest of riches are children…born of
you…kids to have and to hold!

From the poem TWO DOORS (p.30)

As I was writing this book I imagined that if I would be able to select only two people to read it I would choose the mother and father in a crisis pregnancy situation. I dedicate these words to you and your unborn child. In my opening poem, your child will speak directly to you!

We pro-lifers celebrate that Roe v. Wade has been reversed! But that would not stop abortions because states could design their own laws. **Besides saving lives, the most important thing we can do is educate mothers in crisis pregnancies about the dangers they face to their physical, emotional and spiritual health if they have abortions.** That is my focus. In addition, we need to encourage all who have a friend or loved one in a crisis pregnancy situation by either personally to volunteer with the words, "I will stand by you." or help someone else to do so.

The apostle Paul adds, *"The Lord's servant must not be quarrelsome, but kind to everyone, able to teach, patiently enduring evil, correcting his opponents with gentleness. God may perhaps grant them repentance leading to a knowledge of the truth, so they may come to their senses and escape from the snare of the devil, after being captured by him to do his will"* (II Timothy 2:24-26). (See a description of Satan's character (p.101-102)

PRE-READING SURVEY:

Which of these categories are you?
__ I am pro-life
__ I am leaning towards being pro-life
__ I am pro-choice
__ I am leaning towards being pro-choice
When you finish reading this book, please retake this survey and email me the results.

PROLOGUE

Richard Wurmbrand said, "Points of view are points of blindness." Before we accept the opinion of abortion providers about abortion being "safe," let's examine the facts and objectively consider other points of view. I'll report. You decide.

Martial arts experts explain that there are three approaches to competing in karate. First, the fighter can come out with high energy and take a strong offensive, seeking to overpower the opponent for a swift victory. Second, the fighter can play defense, letting the opponent wear himself out, then when the opponent is tired, go in for the kill. But the most dangerous approach occurs when the karate fighter does not commit himself, but rather studies the opponent seeking a weakness, then instead specifically attacks his opponent at his weakest point. What is the weakest point of our pro-choice friends?

I am intentionally taking the third approach. Momentarily I will reprint for you a quote from the Planned Parenthood web site. In it they put up a questionable claim that abortion is "safe and legal". **I see myself as a poet-philosopher.** My goal is to increase your love for life and the beautiful mothers facing a crisis pregnancy. By alerting pregnant mothers to the physical and psychological dangers of letting an abortionist forcibly enter their wombs and take the life of their innocent unborn child, they are needlessly exposing themselves to unnecessary medical and psychological risks. An ounce of prevention is still better than a pound of cure. Thank you for walking arm and arm with me through the door marked life.

One purpose of my writing this book is to evaluate the validity of claims like the following made by abortion providers. **I hope that the discussion that I lay out will help women who are considering an abortion to determine whether or not abortion is safe for them.**

Planned Parenthood, America's largest abortion provider discusses: "DOES ABORTION HAVE LONG-TERM SIDE EFFECTS?" (1/17/2020). "In-clinic abortion procedures are common and effective, and millions of people have gotten these abortions safely. Unless there's a rare and serious complication that's not treated, there's no risk to your future pregnancies or to your overall health. Having an abortion doesn't increase your risk for breast cancer or affect your fertility. It doesn't cause problems for future pregnancies like birth defects, premature birth or low birth weight, ectopic pregnancy, miscarriage, or infant death. Serious, long term emotional problems after an abortion are rare, and about as uncommon as they are after giving birth. They are more likely to happen in people who have to end a pregnancy because of health reasons, people who do not have support around their decision to have an abortion, or people who have a history of mental health problems. Most people feel relief after an abortion. There are many myths out there about the effects of abortion. Your nurse or doctor can give you accurate information about in-clinic abortion side effects, risks, or any other concerns you have."

(For abortion providers writing future descriptions of what they do, a truth from Meister Eckhart, "Only the hand that erases can write the true thing.")

CHOOSE LIFE will document that abortion is not safe. Therefore it should not be legal.

We will be discussing:
Stages of fetal development
Types of abortions
How people can adopt a child
Spiritual dangers of working in the abortion industry
Key abortion statistics
Helpful resources available to those experiencing a crisis pregnancy
Medical problems such as breast cancer, infertility, being unable to carry a child to term, ectopic pregnancy
Psychological problems such as post abortion syndrome (PAS), chemical and alcohol dependency, anxiety, anger and depression, the inability to fully enjoy the pleasures of normal sex, suicidal tendencies
We will graciously accept legislation which permitted taking the life of an unborn child if it is necessary in order to save the physical life of a mother.
We will encourage mothers to view their baby's ultrasound and listen to their heartbeat.

I will share my poet-philosopher's point of view on the sanctity of life. Upon reading this book, if you are working in the abortion industry, I offer my friendship and encourage you to follow the growing numbers of ex-abortionists and become a champion for life. https://abortionworker.com/

Josh McDowell, who has spoken live to more college and university students than anyone in the world, told a true story about an atheistic college professor who challenged Christian students in his opening lecture. The professor asked, "How many of you believe the Bible to be true and relevant to people today? Stand up." The professor walked over to one of the young men standing and ridiculed him by saying, "I have read the Bible and it doesn't make any sense. It is irrelevant. What do you say about that?" The young man looked back over his shoulder at other Christians who were standing, grinned at them, then turned and told the professor, "With all due respect sir, the Bible is God's love letter to his children. Of course it didn't make any sense to you. That's what you get for reading other peoples' mail."

A certain defiant, self-willed and opinionated teenager heard about a very wise elderly man who could correctly answer any question. He plotted a way to prove this man was wrong. He carried a baby robin which had fallen out of his nest up to the home of the wise man and knocked on the door. He asked, "Is this bird dead or alive?" If the man said the bird was dead he planned to put it on the ground and let it run away. If the man said the bird was alive he planned to crush and kill it proving the man had made an incorrect statement. **The wise man looked at the young man sadly, touched his shoulder gently with his left hand and said, "The baby bird's life is in your hands."** (A Gallup poll taken of Americans during 2018 said those who were pro-choice and pro-life were tied at 48%, with the rest undecided).

C.S. Lewis wrote, **"Our choices make us into different people than we were before." (We pro-lifers have nothing to hide. Our pro-choice friends could be more transparent.)**

Jesus took a little child and had him stand among them. Taking him in His arms, He said to them, *"Whoever welcomes one of these little children in My name welcomes Me"* (Mark 9:36,37b).

On September 19, 2019, at the My Pregnancy Choices "Becoming and Belonging" fund raising banquet in Lakeville, Minnesota, Bishop Andrew Cozzens was asked to open the gathering with some remarks. He said, "One poor woman could not afford to pay for the birth of her child. Fortunately a kindly physician offered to donate his services. As part of the prenatal checkup this doctor was sad to discover the child she was carrying had some severe, life threatening physical defects. Then the doctor told the mother, "So if your baby survived childbirth, your little one would be grossly deformed and never be able to live a normal life. Therefore I advise you to abort your child." Incensed, the woman loudly said, "You're fired!"

A second physician who was pro-life was talking with the first OB/GYN doctor. He told the first doctor, "I will take over the case." The pro-choice doctor then asked, "So who will pay for the expenses?" The pro-life doctor said, "If the child is handicapped in any way, I will cover the cost. But if the woman's child is healthy, you will pay the bill."

Then the bishop added, "And this is why I am here. The poor mother in the story was my mom!"

The bishop was handsome, totally healthy and devotedly a Priest For Life.

The crowd gave him a thundering ovation. There have been too many situations where a mother was told the infant she was carrying had severe birth defects. Then, when the doctor aborted the child, it turned out the child was in fact healthy!

In his book, THE GIFT IS ALREADY YOURS, Irwin Prange told about a member of his parish in New York City whose child had died in the womb. She was admitted to the hospital so she could deliver her dead baby the next day. Prange visited and prayed for her. Nothing noticeably happened. But, thankfully the next day, the child was born alive! Let us pray for each other, lifting our needs to the Lord. Always remember, *"What is impossible with man is possible with God"* (Luke 18:27). (See also Reinhard Bonnke's book RAISED FROM THE DEAD.)

Which of God's commandments does abortion violate? It is the fifth commandment which states *"Thou shalt not kill"* (Exodus 20:16). When Christians, even famous leaders say it's ok to abort children, they are heretics. *"Come now, and let us reason together, says the Lord: though your sins be as scarlet, they shall be as white as snow; though they be red like crimson, they shall be as wool"* (Isaiah 1:18). (When we reason about something it means that there are at least two points of view. We will give our pro-choice friends an opportunity to defend their position.)

A baby in the womb is not just a potential human being but is a human being with vast potential.

*"For You formed my inward parts, You knitted me together in my mother's womb. I praise You, for You are wonderful. Wonderful are Your works! You knew me very well; my frame was not hidden from You when I was being made in secret, intricately wrought in the depths of the earth. Your eyes saw my unformed body. **All the days ordained for me were written in Your book before one of them came to be"** (Psalm 139:13-16). (Maybe the child God intended to bring peace to the conflict between the races in America was aborted.)*

God has ordained that your child is created to do specific things with his or her life. If you want to learn how God will use your child, simply let your child be born and be a good parent. The amazing adventure and unveiling of your child's future is right before you. If you buy a magazine subscription or a new book, aren't you eager to read them? If you buy a ticket to a theater, aren't you eager to take your seat? **Aren't you curious to see how the life of your unborn child will impact this world? Before either you or I were even conceived, God planned that I would have the privilege of writing this book. He also planned that at on this specific day at this precise time, you would be reading this paragraph in CHOOSE LIFE and applying it to the life of your beautiful unborn child.**

"Clothe me with skin and flesh and knit me together with bones and sinews" (Job 10:11).

"As you do not know the path of the wind, or how the body is formed in a mother's womb, so you cannot understand the work of God the Maker of all things" (Ecclesiastes 11:5).

TABLE OF CONTENTS

Come See Him Now
An Adopted Teenager's Deepest Fear
Biblical Case Studies Of People Who Were Adopted
Famous People You Might Not Know Who Were Adopted
How Adoption Is A Positive Choice
Types Of Adoption

PLAN A!
Private Conceits – Vanish!
She Must Be Yours
Invitation To A Dream
With This Ring
Thank God Tonight
Grant Us A Child
Christ Creator
Co-Creating Cuddlers
Remembering
Good Samaritans
Within His Broken Heart
A Father's Prayer
Priceless Mother Love
I Pray I'll Have A Little Brother Of My Own
My Beloved Son
Thank You Lord For Mother's Love

ABORTION WORKERS AND PICKETERS
The Picketer
No 911 To Enflame
Once Is Enough
The Trash Man's Surprise
You Could Have Aborted
Soul Celebration
Your Lifting Love
Just A Salaried Guard

PART 1
CHOOSE LIFE!

I have written this book to those who find themselves in a crisis pregnancy. I wish to address your needs. It has been said, "Experience is the best teacher." But there is not time for any of us to experience everything we need to know as we face crisis situations. So I have written observations I have made from talking with people who have been through crisis pregnancies. They share how having an abortion failed to meet their needs. One pregnant mother decided to observe the mental attitude of those entering and leaving an abortion facility; and also to visit the new born ward in a hospital. I strongly urge you to do the same. Think about your needs today. I sure am. You need to know how many regretted their hasty decision to end their pregnancy at the expense of their child. (If you decide to birth and keep your child, you can later choose to put your child up for adoption. But if you end your child's life, you have no way to reverse your decision.) I also reflect on the experience of family members when the mother either had an abortion or gave up her child for an adoption. I share the thoughts of guards and medical staff who work at abortion facilities. I discuss the physical and psychological dangers mothers take when they buy the lie that there is such a thing as a "safe and legal abortion." This section will have the biggest effect on your health. Beware that the sales staff at abortion facilities will downplay the hidden dangers they plot to put you through.

In 1963 a Planned Parenthood Pamphlet asked, "What is birth control? Is it abortion? Definitely not. AN ABORTION KILLS THE LIFE OF A BABY AFTER IT HAS BEGUN. **Birth control merely postpones the beginning of life.**"

"There is a time to be silent and a time to speak" (Ecclesiastes 3:7).

I AM YOUR UNBORN CHILD

I am your unborn child…
    growing purposefully within the
    sacred walls.
I'm bright. I'm strong. I long to be!

You have the power to nurture me
    while I'm in my first nine months.
Or…by an undeservedly cruel act of
    your will, you can end my life
    and alter your destiny.

Nothing in this life remains constant.
Everything depends on your priorities.
Do not be so sure that you will simplify
    your life by ending mine.

Do not be so certain that you will better
    your existence by catapulting me
    from the womb straight into eternity
    before I draw even one sweet breath!

Another couple made a choice to birth
    you…to let you live.
What if the choice for abortion had been
    made one generation earlier?

You wonder what so-and-so will think
    if I arrive unplanned, unintended.
Perhaps you should consider the Creator's
    views too?

Remember…
    Before God formed you in the womb
    *He knew you.**

He knows me, and He can cause a spontaneous
    abortion or miscarriage if He chooses.
Why not abandon the choice as to whether
    I live or die, to God?**

It seems to me that by your "act of love"
    you've said enough, you've done enough.
Now it's my turn! And the Creator's!

I have a statement to make.
    The best of you is being formed in me.
It's not just me you're contemplating killing
    ...it's you.
It's not just infanticide, it's suicide.

So, pledge to me out loud
    I have ears
    I can hear
    that I shall live.

And, as a seal of your intent,
    select my name
    be I a boy or girl child.
And make the sign of the cross over me
    as I am being formed.

My every cell and corpuscle want to be
    loved and to love you.
Let me love you, please?
Is that asking too much?

(If this poem is read aloud, the narrator should be a child.)

*"Before I formed you in the womb I knew you.
Before you were born I set you apart"
(Jeremiah 1:5).

**According to the New England Journal of Medicine, (July 28, 1944)
"31 to 52 percent of human conceptions end in miscarriages."

Why not let the chance of spontaneous abortions rather than a
"planned unparenting, i.e. willful abortion" be left in God's hands
rather than the hands of a deceitful salesperson for an abortion
service?

(Note: I give anyone who wishes permission to copy and distribute
this poem freely. Simply say it was excerpted with permission by the
author of the book CHOOSE LIFE, Dale Stone. I offer it in honor of
unborn children everywhere).

EXIT DOOR EXPERIMENT

Today you are considering
    if you should birth your child and sing
    sweet lullabies, or should you shun
    your child and have an abortion.

There are two places you must go.

You pull up outside one and slowly
    pick a spot. As close as you can get so
    you can see the abortion clinic's doorway.

The day begins. The staff arrives
No one is giving out high fives.

They seem so curt as they step from
    their costly cars. They don't have fun
    or love their jobs. They're passive and
    the air is colorless and bland.

They are a dour grouchy crowd.
They talk, perhaps a bit too loud.

A woman dressed in nurses' white
    pulls out a flask and sips, in flight.

She's certain no one sees her there.
She looks around her. **There's an air
    of sadness...**

Then at 8:00 AM
    a couple comes. They're bickering.
The woman wants him to come in.
He gives her cash. She kicks his shin.

He drives away, says he'll be back.
She gets sick behind a Cadillac.
Then touches up her lipstick and
    steps through the clinic door.

Another woman pushing forty
    comes with a teen. Perhaps her daughter?
Both look drawn out and tense and sad.
They enter silently. Mom's mad.

The singles and the couples come.
They seem distressed. Unsure.
They're bummed.
Approximately three hours or so...
    after they enter, people go.

The same ones who went in, now leave.
Are these folks glad or do they grieve?
You watch for telltale signs...a smile?
It seems they chose a lonely mile.

No one is happy. Empty arms
    have none to hold. No one to charm.
They don't look at each other's eyes.
Their heads are down. And your heart cries.

You sit inside your boyfriend's van.
The tinted windows shield your hand.
They can't see you. The mood is tragic.
There is no joyful loving magic.

Depressed, you know you've sensed the mood
    around this place that sheds young blood.
Your pregnancy doesn't yet show.
You have another place to go.

It is the General Hospital.
The nursery there is two-thirds full.
You pretend you have a friend
    whose child is there. You enter in.

The mood there is ecstatic! Joy
    surrounds each living girl and boy.
Grandparents gloat. The fathers boast.
The nurses laugh, "Who loves the most?"

Just down the hall amidst pink roses
  a cherished child and her Mom poses
  for "just one more."

You touch your womb and breathe relief.
You've made your choice. Firm in belief
  that "life is best!"
And as you leave you hear above you
  a voice from heaven that says,
  "I love you!"

Do your own research. Study faces.
Your town also has two places
  for unborn kids.

Do you know why Noah was successful? He went against
the opinion of every other father on earth. While they were
liquidating their assets he was floating his stock.

"For the Lord God will help me. Therefore I shall not be
confounded. Therefore I have set my face like a flint, and I
know that I shall not be ashamed" (Isaiah 50:7).

"Let us not grow weary of well doing: for in due season we
shall reap, if we faint not" (Galatians 6:9).

"You have made known to me the ways of life. You shall
make me full of joy with Your countenance" (Acts 2:28).

"Now the God of hope fill you with all joy and peace in
believing, that you may abound in hope, through the power of
the Holy Spirit" (Romans 15:13).

"He that keeps you shall not slumber nor sleep. The Lord is
your keeper" (Psalm 121:3).

MATERNAL FIRE

Last night I met a woman who once
    planned a trip to Greece.
She and her husband dreamed of
    relaxation and release
    from all life's pressures as they lay
    and tanned on sunbathed strands.

Then she said she learned that she
    was pregnant, and the bands
    that should have bound her to God's gift
    which was growing 'neath her heart
    instead were stretched toward distant
    shores and she was torn apart.

Her stomach was upset and she had
    thrown up many times.
How could someone with morning sickness
    enjoy the Grecian clime?
She knew that it was legal to free
    herself from her child.

She got a reading from her husband.
He didn't get all riled.
He said, "Just tell me what you want
    and I'll support your choice."
She said, "I've earned and need this trip."
    He heeded her clear voice.

Their child was terminated and
    their trip went on as planned.
They both returned quite rested,
    and looked fit, and well and tanned.
Yet it was not long after that
    they went their separate ways.
Her knight in shining armor left
    and she was in a daze.

Sometime later she met and loved
    another man, but he

had had three kids, divorced and
then a quick vasectomy.
She told him that she wanted kids.
He promised to reverse
his surgery and give her some.
But after they were wed
he changed his mind! Embittered,
she left him, their marriage bed.

She told me how quite recently,
she chanced on number one.
They took a moment to reflect
on what they once had done.
She told her ex she missed their child
and asked if he did too.
They shared their sorrow and their grief
at what they chose to do.

She asked him why he had not argued,
why he did not fight?
He said that when she told him of
her choice that fatal night
that he'd looked deep into her eyes
to read her true desire.
**He told her he was crushed to see
they lacked "maternal fire".**

Then he confessed that if he'd seen
the "smallest twinkle" there,
he would have been enthused and loved
a child with her to bear.

That single woman's forty now.
Her clock is winding down.
The smile that she once wore in Greece
today's a lonely frown.

So when you talk of ending life
and plan those trips to Greece,
remember there is more to "choice"
than instant quick release.

A few years back she found the Lord's
    forgiveness full and free.
And knowing that she's clean inside
    has brought her victory.
Although she knows within her mind
    her guilt has gone away,
Her heart is filled with loneliness
    that somehow seems to stay.
Her life is plagued with sorrow. As she
    longs for and desires
    "her little one" her eyes brim with
    strong, sad "maternal fire".

Friend, if you have a choice to love
    someone you can't yet see...
"Remember I'm a child", not just
    a "problem pregnancy."
And if your child's been living
    eighteen days or maybe more,
    ask someone for a stethoscope
    and hear my heartbeats' roar.

"A-pit-a-pat!!!" "I want to live!!!"
    Please let me grow to term.
I am alive and growing fast.
    I dream and dance and squirm.
And if by chance there is an ultrasound
    machine nearby, please ask someone to
    let you watch me wave to you. I'll try!
I suck my thumb. I think and feel pain.
My ears work too.
And If you take a minute and you learn how much I grew,
    perhaps you would not hesitate
    to let me live. I'm new
    and different – a blend of love.
My father's genes and yours
    have molded me into a treasure
    waiting by life's doors.

If you won't welcome me into your
   home some weeks from now,
   it doesn't matter. Many childless
   homes each day allow
   someone like me to come and live
   with them... It is an option.
Though I would love to live with you,
   I'd much prefer adoption
   to death by suction, poison or
   an assassin's painful knife.
No matter how you choose, remember
   that I VOTE FOR LIFE!

Some day when you are old and gray
   and helpless, sick and frail,
I'll come to you and share your pain.
   Please trust me. I'll not fail.
Some night your arms may ache to hold me.
   I'll be there for you.

I hold a crayon colored star
   backed with some Krazy Glue®.
The glue dries fast. Where do you
   want this priceless star to fly?
Please tell me now. I wouldn't want
   my gift to you to die.

The thread of life is fragile now
   and is so swiftly broken.
Let's always give each life their choice
   and may these words be spoken...
   "I love you."

*"Remember how fleeting is my life. For what futility You have
created all humanity! Who can live and not see death, or who
can escape the power of the grave"* (Psalm 89:47-48).

*"Children are a heritage of the Lord and the fruit of the womb
is His reward"* (Psalm 127:3).

EIGHTEEN YEARS FROM NOW

Eighteen years from now,
   what difference
   will your action make?

Who will then remember if a cutter
   on the take
   conned you into letting him dismember
   your small child?
Who will then recall if the winter was
   harsh or mild?

Eighteen years from now,
   you could be at a graduation.
Your child could be completing high
   school, deep in speculation
   on whether or not to go to college,
   to soldier or learn a trade.

It all depends upon the choices
   that his parents' made.

Is there really any way you could
   pick the death option?
Would you not rather see your child
   put up for adoption?

One in four prospective mothers
   who sadly abort
   lose their reproductive rights.
Fertility's cut short
   by the one who steals from them
   their products of conception.

View your mirror with mother eyes.
Don't slip into deception.
Eighteen years from now you could be
   at a graduation.
Your child could be completing high
   school with great anticipation.

You are asked to make a choice for
  someone growing within you.
Whatever choice you make, it's one
  you never can undo.

Don't forget, within three weeks,
  your child's heart beat is strong.
A short time later, he or she can
  hear you sing a song.

"I care for you!" you lullaby to your
  loved one unborn.
Your child reaches to touch your hand.
You carry life, transformed...

The time goes swiftly.
Memories etch
  indelibly in place.
**Always choose memories that your child can live with
Soon you'll see his face.**

The Greek word for confess is "homolego". Homo means "the
same as". Lego means "to say". To confess means "to say the
same thing God does about your sin, i.e., that it is wrong!"

THE MOST HOPEFUL VERSE IN THE BIBLE

My father, beloved teacher and pastor, Arnold M. Stone used
to say about this scripture, "The biggest two letter word in the
English language is 'if'."

*"If we confess our sins He (God) is faithful and
just to forgive our sins and to cleanse us from all
unrighteousness"* (1 John 1:9). Friends, go to a clergyman
or a mature believer and make confession. Get absolution that
you are forgiven. Don't jeopardize your eternal future because
you have waited to put off confession and being forgiven for
your sins including the sin of condoning, shopping at pro-
choice businesses, voting to legalize, performing or having an
abortion.

SO YOU'RE GOING TO BE A FATHER

Perhaps you've made a mistake
    and you're going to be a Dad.
Don't run away. Don't duck or hide.
Do what will make God glad.

The Lord can cause spontaneous
    abortion if He wills.*
Miscarriages can happen any time.
Men foot the bills.

You've danced and now you have to pay
    to bring your girlfriend through.
The highest and most crucial act
    is what you will to do.

Accept the fact that life exists
    and concentrate on two.
"Your woman" and "your Little One".**
To your own self be true.

Take your lady to the doctor
    for prenatal care.
Do the most that you can do.
Be all that you can dare.

Get counseling for yourself and for
    your child's mother. Plan
    to meet their needs. There's help
    also. Just do the best you can.

Then God will bless your choices and
    a smile will cross His face.
And you will be supported by
    the Lord's amazing grace.

If there is anything within your
    heart that needs forgiving…
    just lay it on the Lord.
Trust Him for righteous living.

Let all those in both families
　　know what is going on.
Expect the best from them after
　　the first surprise is gone.

Then when you've done all you can do
　　The Lord and loved ones will
　　pitch in and help. **Love always
　　beats the selfish choice to kill.**

*According to the New England Journal of Medicine, (July 28, 1944) "31 to 52 percent of human conceptions end in miscarriages."
**"Little One" is English for the Latin term "fetus".

"But my God shall supply all your need according to His riches in glory by Christ Jesus" (Philippians 4:7).

"Know that whatever good thing any man does, the same shall he receive from the Lord be he a slave or free" (Ephesians 6:8).

"Speak up for those who cannot speak for themselves, for the rights of all who are destitute. Speak up and judge fairly; defend the rights of the poor and needy" (Proverbs 31:8-9).

"But seek first his kingdom and his righteousness, (that is His way of doing things and being right) and all these things will be given to you as well" (Matthew 6:33).

DAD'S REGRETS

I wish that I had never killed
    my child that fateful day.
I wish that in my selfishness
    I'd gone a different way.

I wish that I had wed her Mom
    and given life a chance.
My little girl was cruelly killed.
She never got to dance.

She never got to sing or run
    or play with paper dolls.
She never got to go to school
    and laugh within the halls.

She never got to hear me say,
    "I'll love and protect you."
She never got to hold my hand
    or play with Krazy Glue®.

She never got to meditate
    on God's wise words sublime.
She never got to live beyond a
    couple weeks in time.

She never got to share a prayer
    or cook a man a meal.
Instead there was a vacuum sound
    and terminal pain to feel.

Instead she had her future killed,
    she never had a choice.
She never got to say, "Dear Dad,
    I love you!" with her voice.

Within her reproductive self,
    hundreds of eggs were formed.
I killed not just my little girl.
    Grandchildren died, unborn.*

I cannot undo what's been done.
I can't uncross the line
Beware my friend we all must know.
We live on borrowed time.

Don't take another's precious hours.
Don't usurp other's dreams.
Don't ever think that you've a right
to block God's plans and schemes.

*The eggs in an unborn girl's ovaries are called oocytes. They begin being formed during pregnancy. One egg develops and is released during each menstrual cycle. After ovulation, the egg lives for 24 hours.

TWO DOORS

If you chose to abort...at first you will
  imagine how clever you are.
But as you grow older a sadness
  will o're take you. Two doors are ajar...

Walk uprightly through the one that's marked "LIVING".
  Keep your hand off the door that's marked "DEATH".
There'll be pain if you choose to be giving,
  but in giving it's life that's bequeathed.

The sadness and sorrow of killing
  the unborn is real. Our voice
Comes tenderly to you with reason.
  We pray that you'll make the right choice.

What greater gift could you offer
  than to let someone living be born?
How much better it is now to nurture
  your child than to let her be torn
  Into pieces, be suctioned or poisoned
  by unscrupulous abortionists
  who have sterilized, maimed and killed women.
  They just want you to feather their nests.

A doctor who delivers live babies
  could double his income and more
  if he'd stoop to deliver dead babies
  and toss bags of them on the floor.

So go to a live baby doctor!
  And avoid the abortionist's door!
CHOOSE LIFE! Let your name go on living
  and you'll never be lonely or poor.

The greatest of riches aren't dollars
  or stocks, buildings, silver or gold.
The greatest of riches are children...born of
  you...kids to have and to hold!

The wheel of life turns so swiftly.
   the brief weeks of pregnancy pass.
But for those who destroy their own children
   remorse, tears and sorrows amass!

So resolve as you contemplate killing
   that you'll never take that way out.
Then someday a dear one who needs you
   will run joyfully to you and shout,
"MOMMY! DADDY! GRANDMA! GRANDPA!
   Thanks for loving me!"

"Do not be overcome by evil, but overcome evil with good" (Romans 12:21).

"Do not give the devil a foothold. Do not let any unwholesome talk come out of your mouths, but only what is helpful for building others up…And do not grieve the Holy Spirit of God, with Whom you were sealed for the day of redemption… Be kind and compassionate to one another, forgiving each other, just as in Christ God forgave you…Let no one deceive you with empty words for because of such things God's wrath comes on those who are disobedient. THEREFORE DO NOT BE PARTNERS WITH THEM. For you were once darkness, but now you are light in the Lord. Live as children of light (for the fruit of the light consists in all goodness, righteousness and truth) and find out what pleases the Lord. HAVE NOTHING TO DO WITH THE FRUITLESS DEEDS OF DARKNESS, BUT RATHER EXPOSE THEM. It is shameful even to mention what the disobedient do in secret. But everything exposed by the light becomes visible—and everything that is illuminated becomes a light…Therefore do not be foolish but understand what the Lord's will is" (Ephesians 4:27-5:17).

On a personal note, by sharing the thoughts in CHOOSE LIFE, you are exposing *"the deeds of darkness"* and helping deceived people understand *"the Lord's will."*

RATIONALIZER'S REVELATION

Lord, I can't go through with it,
    this problem pregnancy.
It came at such a terrible time,
Dear Lord, please try to see
    that I must terminate my child.
I know it's not ideal.
But, Heavenly Father, I believe
    You know just how I feel.

I plan on asking for forgiveness
    when the deed is done.
Then, I'll get close to You and
    we again can become one.
Before I leave to have it done
    I think I'll read the Word.
I'm not completely peaceful
    and my heart is really torn.

Beloved Daughter, this is Me,
    your Father up in heaven.
I wish to simplify your task.
A text for you is given.

What was the text this mother found
    in Psalm one and forty-five?

*"The Lord preserves all
    them that love Him…"**

There is no hidden lofty thought,
    elusive mystery.
We need not be perfect or strong.
    Love the Lord. Be free.

*"The Lord is fair in everything He does and full of kindness.
He is close to all who call on Him sincerely. The Lord
preserves all them that love Him (He fulfills the desires of
those who reverence and trust Him); He hears their cries for
help and rescues them. I will praise the Lord and call on all*

men everywhere to bless His holy name forever and forever" (Psalm 145:17-21).

"The Lord is good to those whose hope is in Him, to the one who seeks Him; it is good to wait quietly for the salvation of the Lord" (Lamentations 3:25, 26).

"For I know the plans I have for you, says the Lord, plans for welfare and not for evil, to give you a future and a hope. Then you will call upon and come and pray to Me and I will hear you. **You will seek Me and find Me when you seek Me with all your heart**, I will be found by you, says the Lord, and **I will restore your fortunes**" (Jeremiah 29:10-14a). These are my life verses. I suggest you copy and memorize them.

"Truly as the Lord lives and as your soul lives there is but a step between me and death" (First Samuel 20:3).

"You had my mother give birth to me. You made me trust you while I was just a baby. I have leaned on you since the day I was born. You have been my God since my mother gave birth to me" (Psalm 22:9-10).

WORSHIP

Creating Father, strong and good,
    we bless You for our lives and food.
For health and mercy, love so strong,
    we lift our hearts in joyous song.

Pray take our worship as a gift.
Sonorous praises Lord we lift
    to You with gladness, peaceful joy.
Our hearts with Yours, Lord, please alloy.

All works for good to those who love
    You heav'nly Father. From above
    all good things come, all blessings flow.*
So enter us and help us grow.

Prepare us for our task today.
Please lead us in our daily fray.
Empow'r us, Lord, to do Your will
    until the day when all is still.

Our lives are brief, Lord, and so short.
Please lead us so all may report
    they see You in our every deed.
We pray good fruit and Godly seed.

Pray bless our fam'lies, Loving One,
    and help all those who are alone.
Unite us in the glorious task
    of sharing You. These things we ask…

Through Christ our Lord, our Loving Father.
The First and Last. There is no other.
So God, we bow our hearts and knees,
    and wait for all things, Lord, from Thee.
Amen

"In the beginning, God created the heavens and the earth" (Genesis 1:1).

*"And we know that all things work together for good to them that love God, to them who are the called according to His purpose" (Romans 8:28). Rest assured expectant mothers are called to birth their children. "Every good and perfect gift is from above, coming down from the Father of the Heavenly Lights who does not change like shifting shadows" (James 1:17).

THE MOST IMPORTANT PARAGRAPH IN THE WHOLE BOOK

"At the name of Jesus every knee shall bow in heaven and on earth and under the earth, and every tongue shall confess that Jesus Christ is Lord, to the glory of God the Father" (Philippians 2:10). Study context. **Yes, even those who have died and are in the grave, those "under the earth" will do these things: 1. Physically bend their knees and bow to Jesus. 2. Confess with their lips that Jesus is Lord. 3. These actions will glorify God the Father. Then all of us… no matter what our religious or political persuasion is… will be asked to defend our choices. If we bow to Jesus now we can seek and receive forgiveness for our sins. But if we rebel against Him now, when we bow before Him we will only receive His judgment. See also Psalm 22:27-29.**

Study the authority of those who say it is ok to kill innocent unborn children. The Supreme Court isn't supreme. God is the ultimate authority. Believe this and live under the safety of His laws. Your eternal destiny depends on how you react to this truth written by a former murderer. Even as God forgave Saul for stoning the first Christian martyr to death, so God is waiting to forgive you. (Acts 7:1-60).

PART II
LIFE TRIUMPHS!

HE SAW HIS SINGLE MOM WAS PROUD

A few short years ago
 an unwed Mother made a choice.
She had her son. He thanked her well.
 Just listen to his voice:
"Thanks, Mom, for letting me be born.
 For choosing life for me.
Praise God you loved your interests less
 and chose not to be 'free'.

My goal in life's to make you proud
 that I'm your special son."
He told her that, from time to time,
 Was it all joy and fun?
No doubt she had to struggle.
 Single parenting is quite tough.
No doubt she took some flack and
 sometimes said, "That's quite enough!"

Then one day her son earned his wings.
 A Navy flyer, he.
That Mom was, oh, "So very proud!"
 A joyous woman, she.
Then Saddam crossed into Kuwait,
 to rob and rape and kill.
Our President, George Bush, gave warnings.
 Soon, he'd had his fill.

Troops were assigned, air, land and sea,
 to stand mad Hussein down.
But Saddam doubted our resolve
 and misread Schwarzkopf's frown.
One of the half-a-million troops
 that went to save Kuwait
 hugged "Goodbye" to a single Mom.
 He didn't hesitate.

When duty called, his buddies armed
    his aircraft to the gills.
The carrier stood into the wind
    and shot him o'er the hills
    of Desert Storm's most violent clouds.
    His ordinance hit true.
He and his navigator screamed,
    "Saddam, this one's for you!"

Then, as they climbed and banked for home,
    their plane was nailed by flack.
A thund'rous burst of bloody orange…
    too late now to turn back.
Two men were lost that fateful flight.
    One had a single Mom.
"I'll make you proud of me!" he'd vowed.
    She woke up with alarm.

When late that night her doorbell rang
    she was not too surprised.
"Your son's shot down, M'am. We regret
    to tell you." Paralyzed,
    she bid the chaplain and his aide
    to sit down for a spell.
Beneath her outward calm this Mom
    slipped swiftly into hell.

At last they left. Things happened fast.
Draped casket. Bugled taps.
She kept it all inside her heart
    and slept in fitful naps.
Then, when the war was over,
    she chanced on another vet.
A Navy nurse, who rode the oily
    Gulf seas…those two met.

This single Mom, who'd stuffed her grief
    let everything come out.
The nurse wept with her. Held her close
    and let the sadness shout.*
Cautiously, with shaking shoulders,
    memories tearful task.

The best thing that she'd ever done?
    Do you really have to ask?

One day, a few short years ago,
    an unwed mother made a choice.
She loved her son. He thanked her well.
    Now she recalls his voice,
"Thanks, Mom, for letting me be born,
    For choosing life for me!
Praise God you loved your interests less
    and chose not to be 'free'.

My goal in life's to make you proud
    that I'm your special son."
He'd told her that from time to time.
    His victory now was won.
Two single mothers hugged and wept.
    A flyer in heaven looked down.
He saw his single mom was proud,
    saluted, and was gone…

"Life is not measured by its duration. It is measured by its donation."
Scottish born immigrant, Peter Marshall, former United States Senate Chaplain

*The nurse served on the hospital ship named COMFORT during Desert Storm.

"Greater love has no man than this, that he gives up his life for his friends" (John 15:13).

HE WAS NOT GOOD AT TENDERNESS

In tenderness he reached for her.
    He sensed she loved him so.
How could he ever live without her?
    He'd never let her go.

She slept now beside him. The Dawn
    illuminates night air.
He always woke up first and liked
    to contemplate her there.

He recalled when he first saw her.
    He thought, there was no way
that he could win so fine a one.
    Yet she was his that day.

They lived in separate worlds,
    though they shared the
    same name and home.
They knew not how to speak their
    love and both felt so alone.

She conceived first, then married him,
    they did the noble thing.
He always only loved his wife…
    cherished his wedding ring.

He was not good at tenderness.
    This man worked with his hands.
Thick callouses were on his palms.
    His arms were steel bands.

Sometimes when work was slow
    and he was waiting by the phone.
He'd spoken harshly. Frustrated,
    she'd left him there alone.

He loved the way she looked at him
    and cooked for him and such.
What would he do if she should die?
    He needed her so much.

A few weeks earlier, they'd learned
    of cancer in her breast.
He felt as if the lump were his.
    It was so hard to rest.

He never had a way with words.
    He felt sort of tongue tied.
What would his life alone be like
    if his Beloved died?

Sometimes when she was deep asleep,
    he'd reach out with his hand
And use the backside to brush her cheek.
    It was not rough. He planned.

Each day, he thought and sometimes prayed
    how he might show his heart.
He was not good at tenderness
    and knew not how to start.

"Better is open rebuke than love that is hidden" (Proverbs 27:5).

MY TROPHY DATE

Oh trophy date, will you be mine?
I'd love to see you all the time.
I wish I may, I wish I might
    be with you each and every night.

I see the Lord shine in your eyes.
I wish that you would realize
    I'd love to bless you, share things too.
I'd love to spend my life with you.

I know your Mom is single and
    she never got a wedding band.
To me this means she loved you so,
    she never ever'd let you go.

I give your Mom and you respect.
I never would our love neglect.
I wish I may and pray I might
    have a date with you tonight.

TO MY SON ON HIS 18TH BIRTHDAY

My son, you're eighteen now, a man.
No longer will I hold your hand.
You must stand straight and tall, be wise.
You must be diligent, surmise
    what's right, what's wrong
    and choose what's best.

You'll never be like all the rest,
    pursuing mediocrity.
You'll want what's highest. You will flee
    from easy options, go for all
    life has for you. The Lord has called
    you to a life of righteousness.

When you were young, I would caress
    you in your mother's womb and pray
    that every night and every day
    you'd live for God, be pure and strong
    and know how to sing Jesus' song.

Songs are not only sung with words.
There is a melody which fords
    the rivers of the heart and mind.
It splashes down from lofty climes
    of mountain top experience.

The song knows average days of dreariness.
The song knows sorrowful nights of stress.
The song knows when to beg, confess
    forgiveness. No one's perfect, son.

Forgive me for the wrongs I've done
    and for the things I didn't do.
Each day, son, more depends on you.
This is as it should be now.

Learn what you do best, and plow
    a furrow straight and deep and true.
Son, cultivate your field of dreams.
Each thought, each wish, each action seems
    quite unrelated. But they're not.

Each moment follows sure. You've bought
    a reason for all that you do.
Determine standards and be true
    to your self, your family, land
    and Lord. Be real. Understand
    the implications of each seed
    that you tuck in your dream field, son.

Then as life's seasons each are done
    you'll look back with joy and peace.
You will not be sad that you
    avoided what was not just and true.

First cultivate. Then plant your dreams.
And God above will send clear streams
    and rain and sunshine, pleasant rays
    of warm delight. May all your days
    be filled with hope, love, peace and joy.

"Lord, thanks for lending me this boy
    and that my son today's a man.
Reveal Your dreams to him I pray.
      Amen."

Then Jesus told his disciples, *"If any man will come after Me,
let him deny himself, and take up his cross and follow Me. For
whoever shall save his life shall lose it and whoever shall lose
his life for My sake shall find it"* (Matthew 16:24-25).

WE CELEBRATE YOUR BIRTH DAY

As you look to the future
    you know you'll abide
    in the will of the Savior
He'll be by your side.

Your hairs are all numbered
    and so are your days.*

'Cause before time began
    the Lord planned your ways.

Each encounter was part of
    His masterful plan.
You are special to Him
    and to all your fans.

As you live for Him while
    you serve those who are needy
    and share Him with those
    who are hurting or weary.

May your sights stay on Jesus
    Whom you have adored.
May your dreams, thoughts and actions
    show Him as your Lord.

As you look to another year,
    may all your surmises
    be pleasant and joy filled
    with blessed surprises.

So this day as you hope in
    the One Whom you follow,
    may God's highest promises
    overflow your tomorrows.

*"Indeed, the very hairs of your head are all numbered...whoever acknowledges me before men, the Son of Man will also acknowledge Him before the angels of God. But whoever disowns me before others will be disowned before the angels of God" (Luke 12:7-9).

SIMPLE MATHEMATICS

I used to wonder, "Will we ever
    stop abortion's tide?"
I viewed champions like Wattleton*,
    and I was stupefied.

They frankly seemed quite brilliant,
    sharp and smooth, "Devil-may-care."
The ones who spoke out strong for choice
    seemed suave and debonair.

We pro-life folks are often common,
    unpretentious, plain.
And few of us have credentials
    listed after our names.

Then recently, I had a thought that
    gives me certainty.
We pro-life people will prevail.
    We'll have the victory.

The reason is not mystical nor
    couched in deep semantics.
It's clear and plain. A matter of
    simple mathematics.

Most pro-choice people kill their kids.
    The pro-life give theirs life.
Eventually the ballot boxes will
    end all deadly strife.

Each year the pro-life kids escape
    the "pro-choice holocaust."
Eventually we'll o'erturn "Roe!"
    Our flag will top the mast.

So you who are pro-life please fall
    in love. Raise lots of kids.
Each child will one day vote for life.
Abortion's on the skids.

45

Time will rule out. The dead can't vote
　　from garbage bags and drains.
The pro-choice people kill their chance
　　and derail their own trains.

So vote for life by marrying and
　　giving life a chance.
Let's bid farewell to infant death,
　　　Choose life, love and romance!

*Faye Wattleton, President of Planned Parenthood from 1978-1992, ironically she is black.

"A son honors his father, and a servant his master" (Malachi 1:6). (See also Matthew 24:45-51.)

Part III
GRACE TO YOU!

WE KNOW YOUR PAIN:
THE PHANTOM CHILD

Pretend your child is in your arms.
He coos at you with all his charms.

Imagine his unique beauty.
He tugs at Grandma's hand knit booty.

He stops for air and smiles at you.
You are at peace. The skies are blue.

You are responsible and strong.
You did what's right and shunned the wrong.

You are a woman. Keen of mind.
You've chosen wisdom. You're not blind.

Your breasts are filled with love and joy.
You're nursing your own baby boy.

Then you drift from repeated dreams…
        and hear your child's last silent screams.

You look. Your breasts are empty. Bare.
There is no child nestled there.

The price of freedom advertised
        seemed oh, so small. It tantalized.
No one in all the whole world knew
        what you and your lover chose to do.

Now you're alone. You've time to think.
You see the truth. Your spirits sink.

Once you were pregnant. You never sought
a counselor. You felt so caught.

Trapped in a problem pregnancy.
You didn't reach out then, you see?

Why not reach out to others now?
Let friendly women show you how
     you can go forward and forgive.
You can be whole. Be free. And live!

We share a sad, but common bond.
We too reached for the magic wand.

We had abortions. We too felt shame.
We know the crush of guilt and blame.

We offer you a listening ear.
Let's grieve and share a common tear.

You can find meaning in your pain.
With us, you'll learn to live again.

Come now. Don't waste another day.
We offer safety. And a ray of hope!"

*"Where there is no counsel, the people fall; But in the
multitude of counselors there is safety"* (Proverbs 11:14).

"Bear one another's burdens and so fulfill the law of Christ"
(Galatians 6:2).

*"By this all men will know you are My disciples, if you have
love one for another"* (John 13:35).

A REGAL BRIDE

A regal bride, a royal bride,
  comes hesitantly toward God's side.

Assaulted by past failures and
  a windblown house
  once built on sand
  that fell on her amidst much pain,
  she stretches out her hand again
  and beckons to her loving Lord.
'Tis Him she seeks and has adored.

Beside her stand her lovely girls,
  dressed all in white.
Bright eyed, with curls.

They join their mother in the aisle.
Within His eyes they see a smile,
  a tender comprehensive glance.
They realize that it's not chance
  that brought them to
  this day in time.

Awestruck by Him, three ladies mime
  a hesitant, "Hello." How fine
  they look to Him! He runs to them,
  embraces them in one huge hug,
  and they're forever safe.

*"Everyone then who hears these words of Mine and does
them will be like a wise man who built his house on the rock.
And the rain fell, and the floods came, and the winds blew
and beat on that house, but it did not fall, because it had been
founded on the rock. And everyone who hears these words of
Mine and does not do them will be like a foolish man who built
his house on the sand. And the rain fell, and the floods came,
and the winds blew and beat against that house, and it fell,
and great was the fall of it"* (Matthew 7:24-27).

RESTORATION

I am like a David, Lord.
Can You use me now?
Sometimes I've succumbed to things
    that You do not allow.
I've been weak in times past, Lord.
Will You be forgiving?
I choose to repent and change,
    so I can start new living.

I am like a David, Lord.
My passions have flowed strong.
Now I want to live for You and
    right all that was wrong.
Send Your mighty Spirit
    to convict me in this hour.
Take my every longing, Lord.
And change me by Your power.

I am like a David, Lord.
You restored his life.
Can You do the same for me
    and end my inner strife?
I'd love to be useful, Lord.
Have You work for me?
Please dispatch Your Spirit now,
    and grant me victory.

I am like a David, Lord.
You redeemed his soul.
Can I once more please You, Lord.
Will You make me whole?
Let all of my motives bring
    approval in Your face.
Henceforth may each action
    complement Your saving grace.

"And I will restore to you the years that the locust hath eaten"
(Joel 2:25).

*"Restore to me the joy of your salvation and grant me a willing spirit,
to sustain me"* (Psalm 51:12).

SWEET COMMUNION

Sing a song of sadness,
    sing it softly to the Savior.
Taste and see the Lord is good,
    His mercies deeply savor.*
Come and eat the Body of
    the blessed Lamb now broken.
Come all you who are forsaken,
    who no more are hoping.

Come all you whose dreams are dashed
    in tiny fractured pieces.
Come and feel the Savior's love,
    'tis He alone releases
    all the deepest agonies
    within your toiling spirit.
Listen to the Savior sing…
    Be still…and clearly hear it.

"Come away with Me beloved,
    leave the earthly clamor.
Come up on the mountaintop,
    pass through your steel slammer.
Come up where gold meadows melt
    orange, yellow, fragrant flowers,
Swaying gently – let My words
    bring restorative powers."

"Let the breeze of cool winds waft
    away your doubts and fears.
I will take My handkerchief
    and wipe away your tears.
Come up from among those who
    would hinder you from growing.
Place your doubting fingers in My palms,
    the deep scars showing."*

"Come and feel the love marks where
    the Roman spear was driven.
Come experience My mercies,
    dew fresh, sent from heaven.

Come and rest your weary head
upon My waiting bosom.
Let me hold you firmly, still now,
it's you I have chosen."

"You with such a heavy burden
pressing on your shoulders.
You who have steep hilly fields
filled up with many boulders.
Let Me take the stones away
and make your soil perfect.
Let Me place My shield in front
of you so you can deflect
all the flaming darts of him
who'd damn all men forever.
At the mention of My Name
all demons hide and quiver.
Take My Body and my Blood.
I love to be forgiving.
Then walk within the light of love.
Experience righteous living."

Jesus, Savior, Warrior, King
we take Your sweet communion.
This is our time. Cleansed and whole,
together we're forgiven.
Praise the Father, praise the Son
and praise the Holy Spirit.
We believe Your promise Lord!
Let all creation share it.

Your Body makes our lives brand new,
shared joy replaces pain.
Your Blood poured freely on our sin
eradicates the stain.
In remembrance of You, Lord,
we receive Your Body.
We take the cup of covenant.
Your Blood makes us holy.

Praise the Father, praise the Son
  and praise the Holy spirit.
Send us out now to proclaim,
  "Christ died to give us merit."
Praise the Father, praise the Son
  and praise the Holy Spirit.
We worship and adore You, Lord.
  Let all creation hear it!

(Note: one way this poem can be used is as an alternative communion liturgy. Various parts are assigned to the one leading the service, to Jesus, and the congregation. If you mention, "This poem is excerpted from Dale Stone's book CHOOSE LIFE and is used with permission", you may freely copy and use this poem.)

*"Taste and see the Lord is good" (Psalm 34:8).

Jesus said to Thomas, "Put your finger here and see My hands" (John 20:27).
(See also Psalms 22:16, Ephesians 6.)

What are the parts of prayer?

    A Adoration
    C Confession
    T Thanksgiving
    S Supplication: Repeated requests for yourself
    I Intercession: Requests for others

DREAM GIVER

Talk about the love of Jesus.
    Share His blessed Word.
Tell your family, friends and neighbors
    what you've seen and heard.

Trust the Master to reveal
    what you need to pray.
As you intercede you'll feel
    what He'd have you say.

Lean upon the Spirit's wisdom.
Keep your soul attuned.
He's the One Who formed and knew you
    from your mother's womb.

Trust the Lord with all your problems
    even though it seems
    like your way is never easy...
He'll give you your dreams.

"Before I formed you in the womb I knew you. And before you came out of the womb I sanctified you..." (Jeremiah 1:5).

*"Now unto Him that is able to do exceeding abundantly above all that we ask or think, according to the power that worked in us, **to Him be glory** in the church and Christ Jesus, **throughout all generations, evermore.** Amen"* (Ephesians 3:20, 21).

"For I am not ashamed of the gospel, because it is the power of God that brings salvation to everyone who believes: first to the Jew, then to the Gentile" (Romans 1:16).

When Jesus was alive, people didn't dine sitting on chairs with their feet under a table. They reclined on the floor leaning on a pillow which was under their left arm pit. Their feet were stretching out into the room. Furthermore, sometimes and this was one, people not invited to eat could stand along the wall of the dining room and watch and listen to the conversation of the guests. Mary Magdalene was one of the people standing along the wall watching Jesus eat the food the servants brought. Look carefully. At a certain moment motivated by love and appreciation for His forgiveness she stepped towards Him.

ANOTHER LOOK AT THE WOMAN

She did not talk. She did not pray.
She stood behind Him on that day.
Her long black hair, dark Hebrew eyes
    had oft' helped some man realize
    a sinful hour…a stolen act.
She stood there. She could not retract
    from her black past. Her head was bowed.
Remorse spilled down and she avowed
    to leave Him there. She did not wish
    her eyes to show…and yet tears flowed…
    stained seamless robe His mother sewed.
Her makeup ruined, she could not bear
    that He would turn and see her there.
Her priceless gift was nothing now.
She wanted Him, not knowing how
    His mercy worked. A heavy tear
    splashed on His foot. It slashed with fear
    right at her heart. She had not meant
    to ruin His meal. A strong lament
    came to her soul.
She searched the folds…
    the sleeves…the whole of her best robe.
There was no cloth half good enough
    to wipe His feet. My, life is rough.
She knelt down on her knees in shame…
    and then **remembered her long train**
    of raven black, clean glist'ning hair.

And she wiped Jesus' feet right there!
It was not planned...this beauteous act...
She meant no harm. And that's a fact.

So she knelt weeping. Cleansed His feet
    while He reclined there, taking meat.
Next thing she knew, she had her jar
    of alabaster ointment.

Far into the past her mem'ry went...
She heard a prayer her mother sent,
"May my girl always bring the part
    of her that means the most...impart
    to You, Jehovah, what is best
    within her...Help her meet each test..."

The best? Who was she now? A whore!
Who had to sneak to clear the door
    of Matthew's house.
But there she was. Her tears flowed free.
Her sobbing shoulder touched His knee.

The truest longing in her breast
    was to please Him. You know the rest.

(As recorded in Luke 7:38-50).

*"Do not withhold good from those who deserve it when it's in
your power to help them"* (Proverbs 3:27).

*"No good thing will He withhold from them that walk along His
path (in Integrity)"* (Psalm 84:11).

*"Delight yourself in the Lord and He shall give you the desires
of your heart"* (Proverbs 37:4).

*"I love the Lord, because He has heard my voice and my
pleas for mercy. Because He inclined His ear to me, therefore
I will call on Him as long as I live"* (Psalm 116:1-2).

"I wisdom, dwell together with prudence; I possess knowledge and discretion...By Me kings reign and rulers issue decrees that are just...I love those who love Me, and those who seek Me find Me...I walk in the way of righteousness, along the paths of justice, bestowing a rich inheritance on those who love Me and making their treasuries full...but whoever fails to find Me (wisdom) harms himself. **All who hate Me love death"** (Proverbs 8:12-36).

Do abortionists think that God will hold them accountable? What should righteous people do when they learn evil people have power? Be passive? *"Arise, LORD! Lift up your hand, O God. Do not forget the helpless. Why does the wicked man revile God? Why does he say to himself, He won't call me to account? But you, God, see the trouble of the afflicted; you consider their grief and take it in hand. The victims commit themselves to you; you are the helper of the fatherless. Break the arm of the wicked man; call the evildoer to account for his wickedness that would not otherwise be found out"* (Psalm 10:12-15).

In their wisdom, one way abortionists kill the unborn is by crushing them. *"And if you spend yourselves in behalf of the hungry and satisfy the needs of those who are crushed, then your light will rise in the darkness, and your night will become like the noonday sun"* (Isaiah 58:10).

Of the 4 million American children who are born each year, only about 18,000 are voluntarily relinquished for adoption (Source: The Atlantic, October 2021).
There are approximately 117,000 (of the 400,000 in foster care) currently waiting to be adopted (Source: Adopt Us Kids).

PART IV
ADOPTION OPTION!

Finding oneself with an unexpected, unwanted pregnancy (especially when young or single) can be one of the most difficult moments a woman will ever face. Because "safe abortion" represents a relatively "swift" and supposedly "simple" resolution to an unplanned pregnancy, carrying a baby through birth and completing an adoption plan stands as an act of extraordinary courage and love. *Perhaps no other gesture expresses motherhood in its most pure loving form.*

In the United States today **there are 2 million couples seeking to adopt every year** (Source: americanadoption. com). The number of infertile couples in the United States exceeds one million. Recent advantages in reproductive technology will only help one in five conceive. America's abortion rate drastically reduces the number of children available for adoption. **Increasingly it seems that there are no unwanted children, only unfound parents.** 81.5 million Americans have considered adopting at one time or another (Source: American Adoptions National Office). National Adoption Day is celebrated on November 19, 2022.

One day when they were in a store, a stranger asked if the boys with matching shirts were friends rather than brothers, noting that they didn't look at all alike. The child "of color" said, **"That's because I'm adopted. That's when you have the same family but not the same face."**

In a classroom of six-year olds, one youngster said, **"I know all about adoption because I was adopted."** A classmate asked, "What does that mean?" The little girl smiled and said, **"It means that you grew up in your mommy's heart rather than in her tummy."**

The founder of an anti-adoption group was asked how she would counsel an unmarried teen-aged daughter who became pregnant. She said, "First to keep the baby, second to have an abortion, third to commit suicide and only fourth to put the baby up for adoption." Dr. Marvin Olasky explained the reason for hostility to adoption in a National Review Article dated June 7, 1993. **In order for abortion to be legal and accepted, the unborn child must be seen as the woman's property.** To affirm female autonomy it must not be acknowledged that it is better for a child to live in a two-parent family than with a single parent. Therefore **every happy adoptee is a reminder to aborting mothers of the road not taken.** (Robert Frost wrote about two roads which were before him. He concluded, "I took the road less traveled by and that made all the difference." The road to abortion is advertised as the easy way out. Does your child deserve love or death? The child is innocent!!! **Ask any abortionist what your child did to deserve death.**)

Finally, we encourage select crisis pregnancy services to set up an adoption division. This will boost their income stream.

HOW ADOPTION BLESSED OUR FAMILY

My handsome son and his beautiful wife loved children. Because they were unable to have their own, they became foster parents. One of the boys would bite people. My son put on his leather jacket. It protected him. Soon my son was laughing. Then the boy also began to laugh, they bonded, and things became peaceful. Sometimes foster parents adopt one of their foster children.

One day my daughter-in-law was talking with some girlfriends when one mentioned, "Sometimes you allude to the possibility that you might adopt a child. If you want to adopt a child, open your mouth." Immediately she smiled and said, "We want to adopt!"

Within a month, my son and his wife met a single woman who was pregnant. They hit it off. The young birth mother and father selected my son and his wife to be the parents of their child! The birth mom even invited my daughter-in-law to become her birth coach and cut the umbilical cord.

The night before my grandson was born, I wrote this poem.

SIX-POUND SURPRISE

It's 2:00 AM
I lie awake.
Why can't I sleep
for goodness sake?

Short hours more.
The answer lies
within four arms.
SIX-POUND SURPRISE.

Grandpa Dale

Today my grandson is a happy, healthy grade school-age student. I am excited to add that my son and his wife have given birth to two additional children. God is good! My grandson knows who his birth parents are. Our entire family appreciates the birth parents' contribution when they permitted our family to adopt their son! If you ask my grandson his story, he will enjoy telling you, "I was chosen." This knowledge makes him justly feel special.

God bless all birth parents facing a crisis pregnancy who make the loving choice to place their child in the arms of adoptive parents!

GRANDSON GRANDSON

Grandson. Grandson!
Cuddling with your Dad.
Dad's so happy
 where he once was sad.

Grandson reaching
 up to touch Mom's heart.

Forever threesome
 never more to part.
New life ventures.
Mommy loves Dad more.
He's crazy for her!
Draws all – love's du jour!*

Grandpas – Grandmas
Aunts and Uncles too.
Cousins playing.
Life makes all things new!

God in heaven
 smiling from above.
His prized family
 lavished with his love.

All my love, Grandpa Dale

*Of the day.

A certain wealthy farmer had four married sons but no
grandchildren. At Thanksgiving dinner with the whole family,
he held up a cashier's check for $50,000 and said, "Your
mother and I want grandchildren. Whoever gives us our first
grandchild gets this check. Let us pray." When he finished
praying, he and his wife opened their eyes, and they were the
only ones at the table. The four couples had all gone upstairs
to their old bedrooms.

ADOPTION OPTION

You have an unplanned pregnancy.
What are your options friend?
You could abort your little one
    and cause his life to end.

You could interrupt your plans
    and raise him on your own.
T'would be a disadvantaged life
    to face challenges alone.

You and the father could elope
    and try to make a home.
But there are reservations.
"The time is not right," you moan.

Somewhere across the village streets
    a couple has a need.
They long to have a child to love,
    to hug and kiss and feed.
For various reasons every couple
    can't have kids right now.
They pray for someone to bless them
    with a child. Will you allow
    this couple to create a home
    for your child? It would be
    a safe and loving place to grow
    within a family.

Your legacy of life will prove
    the best choice for your boy.
A man and wife offer their love,
    "A God blessed home of joy."

Grandpa Dale

It is impossible for me to explain how much I longed to be a grandfather. My grandson's birth parents were an answer to our family's prayers. We could not possibly respect and thank them enough!

COME SEE HIM NOW

When you've tried all you know how,
    come to God. And you'll learn now
    why it is you're tangent prone.
Come see Him? The "Word"* has flown
    down the moon streaked starlit sky…
    past the paths the angels fly.

Gloria in Excelsis Deo…
    Christ is born! A bless'd rodeo
    witnessed it. Though it was small,
    His Sacred head breached birth canal,
    ent'ring crying, stretching out…
    reaching for a hand so stout.

Joseph held Christ by His heels.
    and in heaven joyous peels
    of thunder…God in heaven laughed
    midst heat light'ning's flannel graph.
God was now a Father proud.
There on earth, in swaddling shroud
    was God's first and only Son…
    come to earth to make us one.
Christ the Lord was born that night.
Mary smiled by candlelight.
Joseph washed Christ's body small.
Cows and donkeys shared the stall.

Maternity had entered time.
Eternity can now be mine…
Embraced in Joseph's strong tanned arms
    a dark eyed infant boy just charms
    his loving step dad. Mary weeps.

And on the hillside tending sheep
    on what had been a boring night…
The meadows suddenly glowed bright!
And shepherds fell afraid and shaken.
"Fear not good men! Please stop your quakin'.
Messiah's born not far from here.
Come, see Him now…in starlight clear."

So with angelic hosts proclaiming
    the shepherds ran full speed, just aiming
    for the spot where glist'ning rays
    pointed down through midnight haze.
Pirouetting doves and sparrows
    sang with joy through all tomorrows.

Down the hills the shepherds ran…
    leaping walls and kicking sand.
They remembered prophets' tales
    of a Savior…Beth'lem fails
    to excite most visitors…

There had never been inquisitors
    like these shepherds in long coats
    jumping over hedges, goats,
    chasing Jesus' birthday star.
On they ran, through the bazaar…
    past the vital village well
    hast'ning quietly, "Don't yell."

Soon they slowed down by the place
    where the manger glowed. Their race
    totally and swiftly won.
There they beheld God's newborn Son!
Reverently they knelt before
    a smiling Christ. "Please close the door…

It's a rather chilly night."
So said Joseph. All was right.
God eclipsed imagination…
    "Mary! Joseph! Congratulations!"
It was as the angels noted…
Christ was born. His guests just gloated.

God had mercy on us with
    that Holy Night of Jesus' birth.
        Amen!

*In John 1, the Son of God is identified as "the Word".
(See also Luke 2.)

AN ADOPTED TEENAGER'S DEEPEST FEAR

The most emotionally loaded exchange I ever read about between an adopted teenage girl and her mom follows. A certain differently-abled adopted teenage girl could never fully accept her mother's love. **Her mother asked, "I need to understand what prevents you from fully accepting my love for you."** The teenager said, "I hate to tell you but I don't think you really want to know and I'm afraid it would make our relationship even worse." The mother said, "I will risk it, tell me." The girl cleared her throat and explained, "I realize that you don't fully love me because the only reason you and Dad had me was because you couldn't conceive a child on your own." The mother covered her eyes with her two hands and started weeping uncontrollably. The father heard it from the next room and came in and asked his daughter, "What's wrong with Mom?" The girl told her father, "I finally told Mom what's been bothering me all these years. I realize you didn't have me for me. You had me because you were infertile and couldn't have a child of your own." The man was holding his wife and comforting her. He also began to weep. He told his daughter, "Your Mom and I could have had our own children but before we got married we thought about all the unwanted children in this world and decided that instead of having children of our own, we would reach out and make a home for an unwanted child. By bravely revealing her deepest fear, this teenage girl realized she was loved for who she was. Her relationship with her parents was beautifully healed and strengthened.

(One of my goals in this book is to strengthen the bonds between parents and their adopted children. **Most importantly I wish to honor the noble decision of all couples in crisis pregnancies who unselfishly chose life. If this true story brought a tear to your eyes, it is proof God created you with a parent's heart. I affirm that you are a kind loving person!)**

BIBLICAL CASE STUDIES OF PEOPLE WHO WERE ADOPTED

I Kings 3:16-27 King Solomon arbitrates between two women who both claimed they were the parent of an infant. It shows the willingness of a birth mother to do anything in order to benefit her child, even surrendering the baby to another woman.

Genesis 41 describes how Pharaoh adopted the Hebrew slave, Joseph. Joseph was given a position normally inherited by the son of a king. Consequently Joseph's skills in interpreting dreams and administration enabled him to save first Egypt, the neighboring nations, then his own family from starvation.

I Samuel 1:21-28; 3:1-20; 7:15 explains how it was not one of the high priest's own sons who became judge over all Israel, but it was rather Eli's adopted son Samuel, who was given that honor.

Esther 2:5-7 explains how the Jewish orphan Esther, who was adopted by Mordicai, her cousin, ultimately became queen and saved the Jewish nation from being liquidated by the anti-Semitic evil egomaniac, Haman.

Matthew 1:18-2:13 describes how Joseph followed the directions of an angel and adopted the Virgin Mary's newborn son, Jesus. **Joseph was the ultimate step-parent** (Hebrews 4:14-16; John 10:10).

At a certain time when the Israelites were living in Egypt, they became very numerous. The Egyptians feared they might rise up and take over the country. So Pharaoh commanded the Israeli midwives that when a female child was born they should let her live. But if the child was male, they should kill the newborn by casting him into the Nile. The Israeli mother of Moses birthed and hid him. When he was three months old the mother made a wicker basket, covered it with pitch so it was waterproof, and put it in the Nile river where the daughter of Pharaoh came to bathe. She found the basket, realized that the infant was a Hebrew child and took pity on him. The older sister of Moses was hiding in the reeds, approached the daughter of Pharaoh and arranged so the mother of Moses would care for and nurse the infant. When the child was weaned, *"the child grew and Moses mother brought him to Pharaoh's daughter and he became her son."* Genesis 2:10. (A geologist read about Moses' mother covering the wicker basket with pitch. He realized where there was pitch, there was oil. So he went to Egypt, discovered oil and changed the entire future of the region, founding the Arab oil industry.)

FAMOUS PEOPLE YOU MIGHT NOT KNOW WHO WERE ADOPTED

Marilyn Monroe, Bill Clinton, John Lennon, Ingrid Bergman, Nelson Mandela, Babe Ruth, Priscilla Presley, Melissa Gilbert, Jesse Jackson, Sarah McLachlan, Truman Capote, Richard Burton, Faith Hill, Steve Jobs, Eartha Kitt, Edgar Allan Poe, Jamie Foxx, Eleanor Roosevelt, Dave Thomas.*

*Dave Thomas named his restaurant chain after his adopted daughter Wendy. The Dave Thomas Foundation for Adoption is the only public nonprofit charity in the United States that is focused exclusively on foster care adoption. Through its signature program, Wendy's Wonderful Kids®, the Foundation provides grants to adoption agencies to hire recruiters who use an evidence-based, child-focused recruitment model to find loving, permanent homes for children waiting in foster care. The Foundation works closely with child welfare advocates and policymakers, provides free resources about foster care adoption and raises awareness through social media campaigns, public service announcements and events.

Choose Life America, Inc. was formed in Florida in 1996 with the idea to use license plate sales to help fund efforts for pre-natal care for women considering adoption services and to help pro-life pregnancy centers and other life affirming agencies get services to women who needed them. (http://www.choose-life.org/) Let's patronize Wendy's.

HOW ADOPTION IS A POSITIVE CHOICE

For the birth parents: they can be assured that their act of love and obedience will place their child according to God's will rather than man's plan. The percentage of adoption referrals by abortion providers is presently very low. (Call any abortion provider and ask what percentage the mothers who come to them birth their child. Call any pro-life agency and ask them the same question.) It is not uncommon for adoption agencies to have a six year waiting list. Approximately one in four women who have abortions can't conceive. **Some of those in the six year long line of those hoping to adopt had sadly prevented the strong healthy child growing safely in their womb from being born. Unfortunately, some mothers aborted the only child they would ever conceive.** Parents who permit their child to be born and adopted are freed for a fresh guilt free start to live their life under God's pro-life laws. They experience His care and blessing. God can even open the door for them to experience spiritual rebirth (John 3).

Dr. Jean Garton in an article written for Lutherans For Life reports the following: **unmarried mothers** are more likely to remain uneducated, live underprivileged lives, have serious employment problems, to require public assistance, live in poverty, have children with health and behavior problems, have infants who die from injuries, to repeat an out-of-wedlock pregnancy, to be school dropouts and to remain unmarried and live unstable lives. (The complete text of Dr. Garton's article "The Adoption Option" was found on 12/15/2019 at https://www.lutheransforlife.org/article/the-adoption-option/).

By contrast unmarried mothers who make an adoption plan for their children are more likely to finish school, obtain higher education, escape poverty, to not require public assistance, to have a higher standard of living, to devote their energies to please a potential husband without having to rush back to watch a crying needy child, to marry well eventually, to be employed 12 months after the birth and to avoid a second out-of-wedlock pregnancy. Neither mom will have to parent prematurely. Both will be free of the financial burdens of parenting, and avoid being forced into a hasty marriage. If young, each can resume their youthful lifestyle.

For the adopting parents: Their sense of crisis at not having a child is lessened because of the successful adopting process. They know that their new child has been "put into place according to God's plan." It gives them "ownership" of the parenting role and enables them to choose to follow the biblical role model for parenting and family.

For the adoptee: It enables the child who has been adopted to know the love which both his birth and adoptive parents have for him or her. It enables them to experience God's love. (I realize that not all those involved in adoption come from a spiritual background. But I wish to invite everyone to imagine the spiritual possibilities which are theirs as they form a new family.) The security of being in a family also multiplies the child's self esteem.

For society: Society will benefit from the formation and values of this new family. Additionally it will benefit from the existence of a growing child who is given the support and nurture to become a good, productive and patriotic citizen.

An independent project, **"The Embryo Adoption Program" encourages people to adopt the "leftovers" from in vitro fertilization.** (IVF, resource list p.190) They have been called "Snowflake Babies" because, like snowflakes, each embryo is tiny, unique, fragile, and frozen. According to a CBS News Report in January 2019, the exact number of embryos in storage isn't known – centers don't have to report these statistics. One study estimated there were 1.4 million in the U.S. Researchers think 5 to 7 percent are abandoned, though it's as high as 18 percent at some clinics. The cost to store an embryo averages $750 per year. Couples who have excess frozen embryos sometimes make them available to needy people.

Adoption isn't easy. It is one of the most complex emotional arrangements in which an individual can be involved. Yet, of the other options – aborting the child or raising the child as a single parent – **Adoption may be the most child-centered option for those in a crisis pregnancy situation.**

It is a healthy, realistic, and sensible choice for all the parties involved.

Adoption can be an enormously unselfish gift to a baby, not only as a way to give a child a secure, loving, and stable family but to give that child the most precious gift of all - life.

TYPES OF ADOPTION

In an **open adoption** the birth mother is involved in selecting the parents for her child. There are companies which screen prospective parents. The mother describes what kind of family she wishes for her child, she looks at profiles including photographs, etc. meets them one at a time until she feels comfortable with the family she considers most ideal. The birth father also needs to be on board with the decision.

During the concluding part of the mother's pregnancy, some of the adoption agencies arrange for her to get funds for things like medical bills, maternity outfits and if she is in school, possibly help with tuition.

In an **open adoption** the birth mother (and possibly the father) may keep in touch with their child. They maintain a connection. They might be invited to special events as the child grows older. The adoptive parents keep the birth parents updated on the child's life.

The child gets to know his birth parents. He or she feels more secure knowing the situation which led to the adoption. The long term psychological development of the child is enhanced by having a healthy relationship with appropriate interaction.

In a **closed adoption**, once the adoption is completed the details about it are sealed. There is no interaction between the birth parent(s) and their child. Once the child turns 18, requests for updates and even for the birth parents and their child to meet can be overcome. There are individuals and companies who help unite a child and birth parents. But even if both parties are interested in meeting, it takes a court order for them to be in touch.

Laws regarding the relationship of birthparents and their children vary from state to state and nation to nation. In September of 2008 Ontario, **Canada passed a law that all adoptions must be open adoptions.** America is also leaning increasingly towards open adoptions. This model works for my family and we endorse it.

When my son and daughter-in-law adopted their son, they set up an **open adoption** arrangement. When the birth parents come to celebrations, everyone seems to get along wonderfully. Our family anticipates that as the child grows older, he will have increased appreciation for the beautiful decision his birth parents made when they chose life.

As time passes, the sadness will grow for women in crisis pregnancies who decide to steal the gift of life from their infant. And the joy felt by families who choose life will increase. I know that my grandson's birth parents are an integral part of his life.

It is also possible for birth parents to include the child they put up for adoption in their wills. I think this is a beautiful idea. The details about adoptions are designed to give the child the most safe, healthy and happy life.

Birth parents feel the love of their child and their child feels their love. There is a healthy relationship between the two sets of parents and the child.

How do you define a woman or couple who let their child be adopted? *"They are not giving up their child, they are sharing their child."* Their child will not feel less love. Their child will be loved by more people. The beauty of open adoption is that the birth parents can love their child without having to assume the responsibilities for financing and raising him or her. The birth parents can live their lives without guilt and they are respected. The birth mother is unharmed by abortion and most importantly they receive God's eternal blessing.

PART V
PLAN A!

PRIVATE CONCEITS – VANISH!

Each soul indulges in his own
private conceits.
One says, "I'm the happiest"…
another, "I'm the furthest from joy."

And whether gladness or wisdom,
strength or experience is the realm,
many in their conceit claim to have
reached the extreme.

Many trust fully, that none has ever
been on their path ~ to this great
a distance ~ ever ~ at any time.

Perchance if they would stop to see
themselves and lift their eyes,
they would see a brother right beside,
and possibly, even someone,
just a step, or a mile out in front.

Perchance they could see they are
in some way, sort of a family…
and the word, "alone" would vanish,
and with it conceit,
and who knows what all else…

Oh, to share*

* **"Love is sharing."** Grandma Lemke, Alexandria, MN

SHE MUST BE YOURS

Father, you've heard it all before,
Unceasing begging at your door
By me. But God it's urgent now;
Please help at once! I don't know how
To make a choice; and so I come
With hope in hand, and hand gone numb,
I'll not strike out again and choose
A girl I am foreordained to lose.

I have begun to sort my needs,
To mold my wants. And ego feeds
These facts to mind: She must be yours,
Spirit-sealed for heaven's shores.
A Christian who can sense the tone
She is to set when she's my own.
And she must want a family,
That's not for us, but is for Thee.

O sure I'll pray for sturdy son
And lovely daughter, full of fun;
But she would also reach out Lord
To draw your lost and struggling toward
The fold of Christ; to help them see
Not just a cradle, but a tree.
She'll be familiar in the Tome
And must be neat: looks, mind, soul, home.

Why are you smiling, God, up there?
'Twas you made Eve! For life was bare.
And Adam, though he owned the earth,
Like me, knew dull days, few of mirth.
So God, let's stop this history
And pick one out, an Eve for me.

INVITATION TO A DREAM

"Come here Meg and sit a while."
My older Cousin's eyes did smile...
Excitedly she beckoned me
　　to hear her secrets. Willow trees
　　with gently dancing yellows, greens
　　enhanced the magic mood. Soft sheens
　　of liquid sunshine brushed her hair
　　as my fav'rit Cousin shared with me there.

"I've got a special favor, Meg.
I'll tell ya straight, and I'll not beg.
I'm getting married!" "That's great!" I squealed
　　and grabbed her hands...as she revealed
　　how Mr. Right had said he could
　　not live without her...and that she should
　　select the date, and her best friends
　　to share the dream that never ends.
"I've found true love and to enhance
　　our wedding day, would you, by chance
　　be willing to hold my bouquet...
　　and scatter petals 'long the way?"

I interrupted her and said,
"But I'm so young, my hair's so red,
　　my knees are knobby, I've got braces
　　and I don't curve in certain places."
My cousin answered, "I can see
　　your marv'lous beauty 'neath this tree.
You're gorgeous, Meg. You're growing fast
　　and each day loveliness that lasts
　　comes from your heart. Your thoughtful deeds...
　　insightful mind...we know the rifts
　　your hugs have healed...the priceless gifts
　　that make you you.
We only want our closest friends
　　to stand with us. Forget the trends
　　the fads and groupies. None else will do.
My Love and I have chosen you.
We want your presence on our day."

I thought a moment. What could I say?
"You betcha, Cuz!" I wept for joy.
I wasn't special to a boy...
    so far that is. But, if Cuz said
    she wanted me...my face turned red.
My Cousin wiped my freckled cheek
    and I, timid, cautious and meek
    was welcomed, chosen, special,
    "in the wedding!"

WITH THIS RING

Joyous love from heav'n descending-
God's own Spirit, condescending
    came to touch my life with yours,
    op'ning all the unlocked doors.

All is now awaiting us.
Yes, I'm going to make a fuss
    over you. I love you, dear.
Cherish you! Away with fear.

I'll be yours with every sinew,
    all my energy….the venue
    is ripe, rosy. All is well.
I love you – my lips will tell
    you again, and then once more.

I'll look on you and adore
    all I see and sense. You move
    towards my heart and life with love.

Come swiftly, darling, to my arms.
I'll be selfish with your charms.
I want all your hugs and kisses.
You're no longer Miss. You're Misses!

Look, the golden wedding bands
    seal our promises. Your hands
    safely clasped in mine feel right.

I'll protect you with the might
    that the Lord has lent to me.
You are loved exclusively!

I praise the Father for conceiving
    your delightful warmth, believing
    that He'd trust me to be true
    to the one He chose. It's you!

Praise the Son for home and hearth,
  for inventing love and mirth.

Praise the Holy Spirit's power
    for leading us up to this hour
    when we can be truly one.
What a miracle God's done.

You are mine and I am yours.
Close the windows. Lock the doors!
Come swiftly now, such sweet endeavor.
And be mine, my love, forever!

(This poem could be read by the groom during their wedding.)

THANK GOD TONIGHT

Thank God tonight that I can
    touch you softly,
    squeeze you warmly,
    kiss you tenderly,
    that I can feel with you securely,
    share with you openly,
    be with you fearlessly,
    that I can dare to love.

Thank God that I can trust myself to you.

No matter what happens from this
    wedding day forward,
    know that I long for you,
    know that I pray for you,
that your deepest desires may be
    met by my deepest desires,
that your most secret wishes
    might be fulfilled in our
    most intimate sharings,
that your most earnest prayers
    might be answered through
    God's most clear guidance!

And trust Him.
I do. Tonight and always.

(This poem could be read by the bride during their wedding.)
(These two poems may be used during the marriage ceremony
at no charge as long as credit is given that they are taken from
Dale Stone's book CHOOSE LIFE.)

GRANT US A CHILD

Dear God, high up there on
    Your throne,
    we've had enough of life alone.
Grant us a child to call our own.
Bring fruit to seeds that we have sown.

We're selfish to the happy end.
Do not withhold, begin to send
    an answer to our largest need.
We'll follow. Go ahead and lead.

CHRIST CREATOR

The birds of winter flutter slowly
Chilled muted colors flying lowly...
Eating seed, digesting, dropping
    them into the grasses cropping.

Birdsongs punctuate the dawn.
Snow crossed meadows. Newborn fawn.
Ice crushed creeks besieged with bright
    effervescent morning light.

Comes the spring! The birds announce it.
Snow Owl spies field mouse and pounces it.
Melting crystals unsheathe trees.
Children race through slushy breeze.
Puddles ponder black galoshes,
    held high as the bike tire splashes.

Screams of glee all soaked and shivery.
New born colts escape the livery...
Prancing o're short grasses...stopping...
    tasting blades while snorting, clopping.

Watch new lambs who frolic feeding
Ewes can't keep up...playful bleating.
Fragrant breezes. Branches touching.
Comes the farmer, oats for munching.

Christ Creator...hope's horizon.
Flowers flaunt sunrise surprising.
Thus the winter of my heart
    blitzed by spring was forced to part.

New life rising. Sorrows fade.
Turn the garden with your spade.
Plant the rows. Sprinkle with water.
Dance and sing each son and daughter!
Created for God's bounteous pleasure
    giv'n to us with fullest measure.

NOTE: We have established that God created all things. But, what is His attitude towards us? We are created in His image and are also part of His creation. *"The Lord is faithful to keep all His promises and loving toward all He has made"* (Psalms 145:13).

"Hear me when I call, O God...have mercy upon me and hear my prayer...the Lord will hear when I call unto Him" (Psalms 4:1,3).

"He will call upon Me and I will answer him. I will be with him in trouble. I will deliver and honor him" (Psalms 91:15).

"I will instruct you and teach you in the way you should go; I will counsel you with my eye upon you" (Psalms 32:8). (Think about how a mother watches her children playing on the sidewalk of a busy street. She keeps her eye on them and warns them so they don't wander into the traffic.)

"Do not be afraid or terrified because of them. For the Lord your God goes with you. He will never leave you or forsake you" (Deuteronomy 31:6).

"Trust in the Lord with all your heart and lean not on your own understanding. In all your ways acknowledge Him and He will make your paths straight" (Proverbs 3:5,6).

I suggest you make a list of the key concerns in your life. Of decisions you need to make. Don't risk making the decisions on your own. To make the best choices, bring your cares and concerns to the Lord. List also the implications of each choice. Once a mature Christian was asked what he would do if he ever felt unsure about his love for his mate. He said, "I would kneel beside my bed and bring the matter to the Lord. And not get up until I heard from Him. Then I would follow His direction."

"Rest in the Lord, and wait patiently for Him; fret not" (Psalms 37:7). God finishes what He starts.

"But my God shall supply all your need according to His riches in glory by Christ Jesus. Now unto God our Father be glory forever and ever. Amen" (Philippians 4:19-20). **He meets "all your needs."**

"When you lie down, you shall not be afraid. You shall lie down and your sleep shall be sweet" (Proverbs 3:24).

A pastor helped an elderly man who was on his death bed to believe in Jesus. The man said, "I don't know how to pray. How do I do it?" The pastor pulled a chair next to the man's bed. Then he said, "Imagine Jesus is sitting in this chair. Just talk with Him." The man was delighted at this privilege. The next morning the nurses reported that this man had died in his sleep. A peaceful smile was on his face. His hand was reaching out touching the chair.

On a personal note, one of the most exciting times in our marriage was when we decided to have a child and went off birth control. The intentionality of making love to conceive a baby brought unequalled excitement. Our love for each other soared to new heights.

CO-CREATING CUDDLERS

Come to me sweet pregnant woman
    filled with my love, growing strong,
    large and larger. You're a wonder.
How I boast of you, My Song.

Honeyed lotions. Laughing, loving.
Soft caresses. Turtle doving.
Moneyed potions. Stretch marks wand'ring.
Heartbeats steady. Feel his moving!

I can't sleep with you facing me.
Let's be like two spoons.
You first. I following
    warmly now – the back of your knees
    touched by the front of my knees...
Your back and buns snuggled
    by my thighs and chest.
Your skin touching my skin.

Our child nestled 'neath your heart.
Our four hands touching his two hands.
Oh, the wonder of it all. Co-creating!
I kiss your body, claiming it as mine.
Your body is my body. My body is your body.

Our child's body is somewhat our body...
    yet he has a separate blood supply,
    most likely a different blood type than yours.
Most probably masculine protective hands, like mine.
Hopefully a generous, giving spirit, like yours.
Undoubtedly full of mischief and excitement!
A perfect blend formed by the Lord of Life
    with two enthusiastic supporting
    stars at the conception parties.

Lord, have mercy. It feels so good to be expecting!
Majestic movement, mysteriously reaching toward birth.
Let none dare hint that our child is anything but alive,
    full of expectations, talented, exuberantly ours!

"Father God, may each moment of growth
    within the sacred walls be special,
    purposeful, remembered, cherished."
Sweetheart, I am so proud of your maternal fire!
I never wanted, appreciated nor needed you more than now!

With each kiss, as you nestle your tired
    head on my left arm and
    I trace the curve of your shoulder,
    taste the softness of your neck and right ear,
    embrace your femininity in all its fullness.
With each kiss, I thank God that you are
    my Co-Creating Cuddler.

*Even every one that is called by My name: for I have created
him for My glory, I have formed him; yes, I have made him"*
(Isaiah 43:7).

REMEMBERING

Night times are the hardest times
    when no one else is there.
Remembering a child's kiss
    but now...emptiness...air.
Remembering sweet sounds of running...
    giggles...slamming doors.
Remembering the joys of doing
    simple little chores...
Remembering tub toys and shampoos...
    hot towels from the dryer...
Warmed up footie jammies...
    prayers and hugs that love requires.

BOMBERS HAVE EXPLODED
    IN-BETWEEN A PARENT'S ARMS!

Gone are loving glances
    and a mother's needed charms.
Run towards danger...
Help the victims.
Never mind the risk.
Sacrifice of helpfulness
    complete...Won't someone frisk
    dang'rous felons...check the vans...
    explosives riding low?
Tons of bombs make the shocks creak.
How can someone go
    bomb the building?
Bomb the workers?
Bomb the children too?
There are different rules for death...
Life's options are too few.

Who is safe now? Who can know?
GOD PROTECT US? We are tired.
    Please let peace reign strong.
Let the tears and vengeful longings
    be replaced by song.

Give us hope, Lord! Grant us mercy!!
  Send angels on wings
  to protect us all from harm…
  remove the death that stings.

Help us. We long for protection.
Grant us hope in resurrection.
We place all our trust in You.

Lord, create our lives anew.
  Amen.

(This poem was written on April 19, 1995 after a bomb-loaded van exploded destroying much of the Alfred P. Murrah Federal Building in Oklahoma City. The building also contained a child care facility. 168 lives were lost.)

"God, in His mercy and grace is faithful. From everlasting to everlasting the Lord's love is with those who fear Him, and His righteousness with the childrens' children" (Psalm 103:17). Families and especially grandparents who love life make a difference for generations to come. *"People yet unborn praise the Lord"* (Psalm 102:18).

Not only does abortion kill a child, it deeply wounds a woman. Although at first she may feel a sense of relief that her problem has been solved, eventually the reality of this unnatural choice sinks in. When it does, the guilt and shame can be overwhelming. This awful reality can bring the same devastation to fathers, grandparents, siblings and children. **When a child learns that his mother has killed what would have been his sibling, consciously or subconsciously such a child might also be afraid of being killed.** Abortion is not "just an election issue". Because abortion can destroy relationships within families as well as between God and an individual, it is also "a spiritual issue". *"People were bringing little children to Jesus to have Him touch them, but the disciples rebuked them. When Jesus saw this, He was indignant. He said to them, 'Let the little children come to Me, and do not hinder them, for the kingdom of God belongs to such as these. I tell you the truth, anyone who will not receive* *the kingdom of God like a little child will never enter it'.* **And He took the children in His arms, put His hands on them** *and blessed them"* (Mark 10:11-16). Today we bring children to church that we might *teach them*. Let us also reach out and lovingly touch children not only in our places of worship, but as needed, where needed.

GOOD SAMARITANS

Somewhere across the hall or street,
    the night time hears a mother's feet.

She's up to check a child's cry.
She's up to help, to soothe, to try...
    To love.

Somewhere across the ocean wide,
    a child lays hungry, and inside
    his stomach there's an emptiness.
His heart's bare too, no soft caress.
    No love.

Somewhere back in a history book
    a strong young father crossed a brook
    to chase wild animals away.
He told his wife and kids to stay.
    That's love.

Somewhere back in your mind, a thought
    of some kind deed someone had brought
    to you wells up. It's good. It's there
    to urge you now. So live, so share.
    So love!

WITHIN HIS BROKEN HEART

In deep despair…from lonely hours
    of anguish, tears, frustrated powers
    of longing…I reach out and touch
    the tender-hearted Christ.

So much He grieved and longed for me.
So often He reached out, again
    and always opening up His soul.
    in tenderness and love. The whole
    of all He left in heaven above
    defies description. Giving love
    personified in nail-scarred hands.

Reach out Jesus! Let Him share
    the mercies which well up and care
    for all the weeping wounded ones.

If you have pain and sorrow cleaves
    to you like armor…Jesus leaves
    all His own preferences, and grieves
    for you. He shares your sorrow.

He's here today, and on the morrow,
    He'll waken you, refreshed. So sleep
    and know a loving Lord will keep
    each sorrow, hope, each care and dream
    within His broken heart.

A FATHER'S PRAYER

Now I lay my son to sleep.
I pray dear Lord, his soul to keep.
Accept our thanks for little joys
    this day has brought.
    for friends – for toys –
    for laughter – hugs – for shoulder rides
    for having hearts where Christ resides
    for bumps and scratches – fun and tears –
    for hopes that draw us through the years.
Please give him pleasant dreams tonight
    and may tomorrow's sun shine bright
    upon our love.

Published March 1973 in THE LUTHERAN AMBASSADOR, used with permission.

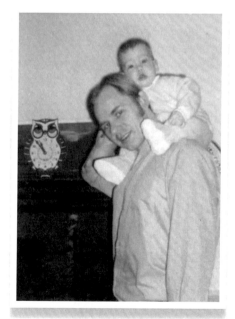

Author Dale M. Stone
with his son. He is 10 months old
in this photo.

PRICELESS MOTHER LOVE

Make me a moon, dear God I pray,
    creating Father mine.
Let me, though inconsistent, weak,
    reflect glory divine.
I bow my robust self and pride
    and kneel in frustration.
I use too many pronouns and
    have caused much consternation.
I come and pause...Please visit me.
    I need Your presence strong.
I humbly pray, let me become a moon,
    to shine Your song
    down on a misdirected world, too keen
    to kill a Star.
They do not know Your Child, who came
    to love us from afar.
We intercept millions of lives
    before they're born alive.
And torture them, so small and helpless.
    Painfully they strive,
Dear Master, may I be a moon
    to educate the world.
May I consistently reflect
    Your light from above.
Dear Lord, may each child that's conceived
    know "priceless Mother love."

"Behold, children are a gift of the Lord. The fruit of the womb is a reward. Like arrows in the hand of a warrior, so are the children of one's youth. How blessed is the man whose quiver is full of them..." Psalm 127:3-5).

"O taste and see that the Lord is good: blessed is the man that trusts in Him" (Psalm 34:8).

I PRAY I'LL HAVE A LITTLE BROTHER OF MY OWN

Someday I hope to have a little brother of my own.
I'd like to hug and play with him within our loving home.
I'd promise that I'd let him nap when he was tired out.
And if he wished to use my toys, I'd share and never pout.

I'd like to show him how to toss a ball and catch a fish.
There are a million things which we could share.
    That's all I wish.

I've heard about abortion and I hope you don't have one.
'Cause if you do, I'll be alone and won't have any fun.

Maybe it's my fault. I don't always mind first time I'm told.
I'm working on being better now that I am growing old.

I think that you're great parents. You did real well with me.
We always have room for one more. On that we must agree.

So, Dad and Mom, please let him live!
    He's welcome in our home.
Someday I pray I'll have a little brother of my own!

Many who choose to abort already have a child who would love a playmate.

MY BELOVED SON

Look up. See the mountains before you.
Challenges beckoning your willing spirit.
Undeterred and excited by the opportunity
    to pit your skills against the rock façade
    you leave the safety of the valley,
    rope up and start your climb.

Joyfully plot your ascent!
Read the rocks.
The path unfolds as you move
    relentlessly upwards.
The sweat of honest effort
    purges the cares of the day.
And you pull on your water bottle.

Glancing downward your joy level
    rises as the eagle soars below you.
Studying the path before you
    you reach for the heights.

He who made the mountains
    sends a warm breeze
    of encouragement.

The weather may not be perfect,
    but the path God has chosen
    for you is.
May you aim for the summit
    buoyed by the prayers
    of loved ones here and
    in heaven.

Cherished beyond your imagination.
Loved always by your parents.

THANK YOU LORD FOR MOTHER'S LOVE

(This song uses the melody from – "Baby Face")

Mother's Day…it's not like any other. Hip Hooray!
Let's tip our hats and recognize that, hey,
    Moms are great…where'd we be without them?
    Let's show love before it's too late.
Mother's Day…thank God He made them and that
    they love us so much. If it were not for Moms
    who sew and fill our tums…
    then life would not be worth a nickel
    …we'd be in a pickle…
Here's to your our Mother's dear!!!

Mother's Day. They love us when we're sweet
    and when we're not.
They're not like normal mortals…what they've got
    is great soul
    hearts and hugs that give us joy
    and prayers that make us whole.
Mothers are the greatest people ever,
    God sent from above.
Sometimes we are cute kids…
Sometimes we're on the skids…
    for them our flag's unfurled.
Thank you Lord, for Mother's love!

Dads love Moms. They bring them flowers and presents,
    make them smile.
Help them around the house and all the while
    they tease them…make them promises
    and sometimes even take them shopping.
Dads love Moms…they even help with mopping.
    carry out the trash.
Our Mom's the world's best. You can have all the rest.
We thank the Lord that she's our Mother.
We can never pick another.
Thank you God for Mother's love!

Moms are great...they say that we're a treasure.
Moms are grand...they love us without measure.
Everyone needs their touch.
They're the ones we love so much
        and even when we're naughty...Moms love us...
They teach us right from wrong.
To them we sing this song...
We celebrate each Mom...and all the things they've done
        to make our life worth living...thank you.
Even when they spank you...
Moms we honor you this day!

We love you Mother. Thank you Lord for Mother's love!

(My mom often loved to wave to young children, catch their
eye and make them smile. I enjoy talking to young children
and saying, "Hello, you have a beautiful smile." For example,
sometimes at places like a restaurant I talk to a family sitting
together as I walk by them and say, "Excuse me, I just wanted
to say you have a nice looking family." I enjoy seeing them
return a smile and thanking me. Try it sometimes.)

PART VI
ABORTION WORKERS AND PICKETERS

Dr. Anthony Levatino started to process lives he killed as an abortionist when his wife struggled to get pregnant. His OB/GYN practice included offering abortions. As he aborted roughly 10 children a week, he silently wished he could take one of them home. Thankfully the Levatinos were eventually able to adopt a little girl they named Heather. Later they had a son. The doctor continued to do all abortions until his daughter, Heather, age five, was hit and killed by a car. He had done over 100 second semester suction D&E procedures on children who were up to 24 weeks of age. **One day he realized that he was acting like an assassin who took money in order to end someone's life**. He was told before doing a fifteen minute second trimester procedure, "Here's 800 dollars. Will you kill my baby?" **We hear all the time abortion is medically necessary.** *He saw 100's of pregnant women with life threatening illnesses such as cancer, heart disease, diabetes out of control, etc. In all those years, the number of babies he had to deliberately kill to save the life of the mother was none.* **It takes 24-72 hours to gradually widen the birth canal and prepare a mother for a late term abortion. In one instance a woman who was late in her second trimester showed up at his practice with a dangerously high blood pressure of 220/160.** She could have had a stroke any minute. **Within an hour he gave her a C section** and the mother and child did just fine. **Had she been forced to wait for an emergency late term abortion, she would most likely have had a life threatening stroke**. *So the solution for a woman who has a medical crisis while in the second trimester or later is to stimulate her child to be born or give her a C section* (I invited specific discussion about his two solutions. If you are an abortionist, what percentage of the time have you needed to kill a child in order to save the life of the mother? If you are considering getting an abortion, ask your abortionist how many times he or she had to kill an unborn child to save the life of a mother. Contrast that statistic with what percentage of mothers died when they were given a "safe and legal abortion?") Yes, some prematurely born children were lost when these two options were taken. But many lived!!

Strong suggestion: **Enter Doctor Levatino Abortion Procedures in your search engine.** Click on "The Story" to view the former abortionist's amazing 25 minute interview with Lila Rose. Lila Rose asked him, "What impact did picketers who sometimes yelled at abortion workers have on you?" He said, "I thought they were kooks. But I had a new patient who came in for an annual checkup and pap smear. Following the exam, she asked, 'May I discuss something with you?'" He realized women like to have a little rapport prior to entering into a meaningful conversation. He replied, "Surely. What can I do for you ma'm?" She said, *"I believe God sent me here to tell you, you were not created to do what you are doing and to stop doing abortions."* Then she politely smiled, thanked him and left. She kept him as her OB/GYN doctor. She used him for her annual checkup and pap smear and even brought him brownies and politely gave him the same message. Doctors care about what their patients think. We in the pro-life field describe what she did was, **"adopting an abortionist."** *Should you research abortionists in your state and strategize to make certain that pro-life women become their patients, adopt them and politely encourage them to stop doing abortions?*

After you finish reading this book, CHOOSE LIFE I suggest you to go back to the website Dr. Anthony Levatino Abortion Procedures and watch the segments in this order: D&E, Aspiration, Pills, Induction. I encourage you to study the descriptive drawings and read his explanation of the various types of abortions.

THE PICKETER

I am just a picketer,
    signed up for today…
Wondering if I should go
    and by my presence say,
"I believe that unborn kids
    have the right to live!
And even if mistakes were made
    it's best to forgive.

Two wrongs never make a right."
That's what my sign will say,
"Let your child live and love,
    nurse, crawl, kiss and play."

Turn around, go home and give
    life within a chance.
Don't get sold on murdering!
Skip their song and dance.

Just because male justices*
    declared that you can kill
    your child when he's in the womb…
    by chauvinistic thrill
    seekers bent on salting out,
    suctioning or worse…
Keep these misinformed men
    from going to hell in a hearse.

Your vote is the only one
    that your child needs today.
"Let your child live and love,
    nurse, crawl, kiss and play."

Are you wondering if you can
raise your child alone?
No one can. We offer help.

*All nine Supreme Court justices who ruled on Roe vs. Wade
were men.

NO 911 TO ENFLAME

Today on "Divorce Court" on TV
   I watched a horrid scene.
The parents of a nine year old
   fought for her custody.

The crucial evidence was on
   A tape from 911.
The girl's voice begged
   "Someone please come...

Please stop my mom from beating grandma!
   Grandma's on the ground!"
The girl was in acute distress
   and prayed help could be found.

The mother was in strong denial
   and grandma sheltered her.
Through quiet questioning the judge
   discovered the truths there.

The grandma finally admitted she
   had taught her daughter, "Pain
   was how one spoke in frustration..."
There was no more to gain.

The truth was out...Mom had beat grandma.
Mom may not have struck her girl.
But generational violence
   had spun them in a whirl.

Before he ruled the judge quoted
   a poem from ancient times.
The key line was, "A child shall lead
   them..."* Truth lives on in rhymes.

The loving father won his girl.
She from violence was taken.
The mother and grandmother wept.
   Their lifestyles were so shaken.

Sixty million children died an
    anguished death of pain.
The problem is, that in the womb
    there's no 911 to enflame
    our indignation.

The child can't call.
So we the loving, band
    to urge that murdering be stopped!
For life and right, we stand!

During an abortion your child's heart-
    beat speeds up in panic, 300%!
It's always true and always tragic
    up through the final day
    of pregnancy, abortion is
    an oft' accepted way
    of coping with a crises in
    reality or dreams.
Too bad there is no 911
    to record infants' silent screams.

However, when abortion starts
    the child thrashes to flee
    the mangling tools and sucking wands.
Soon, death results. Mom's free?

"You do your thing. And I'll do mine.
Don't force your views on me.
In open minded America
    we have this liberty."

But just because it's legal to
    torture and kill your kids
    doesn't make it morally right.
Unscrew Pandora's lids.

Before you have an abortion
    ask to watch one and hear
    the fetal monitor proclaim
    the child's heartbeat of fear.

The lack of laws to save unborn
   are screaming to be changed.
Until they are, manipulated
   women are estranged.

Kept from reality…they dream…
   of things which never were…
They wonder if they'd followed right
   on their blood red detour.

* *"The wolf will live with the lamb, the leopard will lie down
with the goat, the calf and the lion and the yearling together;
and a little child will lead them"* (Isaiah 11:6).

"You shall not murder" (Exodus 20:13).

*"Whoever sheds human blood, by humans shall their blood be
shed; for in the image of God has God made mankind. As for
you, be fruitful and increase in number; multiply on the earth
and increase upon it"* (Genesis 9:6-7).

*"Let your face shine on your servant; save me in your
unfailing love. Let me not be put to shame, Lord, for I have
cried out to you; but let the wicked be put to shame and be
silent in the realm of the dead. Let their lying lips be silenced,
for with pride and contempt they speak arrogantly against the
righteous"* (Psalm 31:16-18).

*"When you give it to them, they gather it up; when you open
your hand, they are satisfied with good things. When you
hide your face, they are terrified; when you take away their
breath, they die and return to the dust. When you send your
Spirit, they are created, and you renew the face of the ground"*
(Psalm 104:28-30).

ONCE IS ENOUGH

One time I bowed.
I can't condone
   denial now.

I flexed my will
   but when cold shrill
   vacuuming sound
   ripped life, I found
   that I was wrong.

Now, no more song.
Life passed through air…
   suctioning death.
No funeral wreath.
I'm plagued with grief.

Once more I'm caught.
Programmed? They taught
   me abortion was not a sin.
Shall I go in…again?

I nearly went inside.
God sent a pamphleteer.

She met me there.
Told me what's fair.

I was not sure.
Should I detour
   from life once more?
One time they tore
   life from my womb.

NO! There is room
   in my life for you
   my child! The door
   to death is closed.
I'll bow to death no more.

I looked. I viewed
   the ultrasound.
My faith renewed
   in life, I found
   that I can live life
   freely now.

And love you,
   mother you
   my dear child.

Satan is the Father of Lies. He likes to con people and get
them to believe that once they make a mistake their life is
over. Proverbs 24:16 blows the lid off that misconception,
promising, **"For though the righteous fall seven times, they
rise again,** *but the wicked stumble when calamity strikes."* We
will be addressing how we can be lifted from being numbered
with the wicked to being transformed and becoming righteous.
Approximately half of those having an abortion have had one
before. No matter your history, be encouraged!

*"Submit yourselves, then, to God. Resist the devil, and he will
flee from you"* (James 4:7).

Tell Satan, "I resist you. Leave me alone." Tell God simply, "I
fully submit myself to You."

In the Lord's prayer we pray, *"Lead us not into temptation,
but deliver us from evil."* This petition can also be translated,
*"And lead us not into temptation, but deliver us from the evil
one"* (Matthew 6:13).

Satan likes to intimidate us and tell us about our past sins,
so we become pessimistic and won't attempt to fight for what
is right. When Satan tells us about our past, we can tell him
about his future.

At the last judgment the Lord will say to those on the left,
*"Depart from me accursed ones, into the eternal fire which
has been prepared for the devil and his angels"* (Matthew
25:41).

At one time Satan had an important position of authority in heaven. But his pride led him to tempt the angels to worship him instead of the Lord. So Satan and 1/3rd of the angels were exiled from heaven. Eventually they will end up in a hell of fire.

Satan has a limited time to tempt and get we who are on earth to sin. The following terms describe Satan:

He is **accursed**, and headed for hell fire Matthew 25:41

He is a **devourer** I Peter 5:8

He is a **liar** John 8:44

He is a **murderer** John 8:44

He is an **accuser** Revelations 12:10

He is a **tempter** Matthew 4:3; I Thessalonians 3:5

He is a **destroyer** Revelations 9:11

He is the **prince of the power of the air** who transforms people into "sons of disobedience" who live in the lusts of the flesh, mind and are transformed into children of wrath Ephesians 2:2

He is the **god of this world** II Corinthians 4:4

He is **"fallen from heaven"** and the high position of being **"Lucifer, son of the morning"** Isaiah 14:12

He is a **coveter**. He coveted being like "the Most High God" Isaiah 14:14 (Satan successfully enticed one third of the angels to worship him. Therefore God cast all of them out of heaven. They represent Satan's army of demons. They have limited power now but will ultimately be cast into the lake of fire along with those on earth who serve Satan.)

He is a **deceiver**. His chief character trait is "deception". He deceived Eve and Adam into disobeying the Creator and eating of the forbidden fruit. Genesis 3 (See also Revelation 20:10.)

He is a **thief** who comes to STEAL, KILL and DESTROY (John 10:10)

THE TRASH MAN'S SURPRISE

I drive a local garbage route
    and do my work quite well.
I pick up papers, bottles, but
    on one day there's this smell.

I grabbed a plastic garbage bag
    and nearly fainted when
    a tiny human leg, an elbow
    and part of a chin
    was sticking out through a small tear.
I chanced a look within.
The dumpster bag was full of body parts
    from kids yet to be born.

They'd never have a birthday,
    nor a joyful Christmas morn.
Some infants were all torn apart
    and some had skin bright red.

I grabbed my stomach and threw up
    and nearly lost my head.
I wanted to rush through that door
    and protest…but instead
    I silently and tearfully
    set them reverently on the floor
    of the passenger seat of my truck.

Note: in various locations body parts of unborn children have been discovered in trash bags. Thankfully some have been turned over to the authorities and given a proper burial.

Search the internet for the name of the abortionist Dr. Ulrich "George" Klopfer. Following his death at age 69, 2,246 preserved fetal remains were found in his garage and another 100 in the trunk of his car. He operated three abortion clinics during his career. He aborted over 20,000 infants.

YOU COULD HAVE ABORTED

It's wonderful not to have children.
They're messy and get in the way.
And when they are infants they cry out
    and control you by night and by day.

They need you to kiss them and hold them.
And if you have two they will fight.
They want lots of toys, food and fun times
    and demand hugs and stories each night.

When you want to sleep in on the weekends
    they beg you to take them to church.
They ask that you pray and sing with them.
Soon they're gone and leave you in the lurch.

Then they marry and it all starts over.
They park grandkids with you and leave.
You want to sleep in on the weekends.
You've worked hard and earned a reprieve.

But these pesky young grandkids need your love.
They demand your attention and dough.
And your kids will be asking for money
    all their lives. You can't get them to go.

They may name their children after you,
    but it's only a ploy for your love.
They pretend to ask for your counsel
    when you'd just as soon they'd go and shove
    off, that is.

You will end up in debt every Christmas
    taking loans for gifts they'll never use.
And to think that you could have aborted.
Good Lord! What did you choose?

All too soon you'll be grey, weak and older
and you may want someone there by your side.
You may lose your eyesight and hearing
and you may need some love or a ride.

And when you are frail and bedridden
and your life here on earth is near through,
You may have a home or some savings
and you'll need someone to give it to.*

And you may wish that someone will miss you
and carry your name on when you're
on the other side of that great river.
Then follow you to heaven's shores.

If you chose to abort...at first you will
imagine how clever you are.
But as you grow older a sadness
will o're take you. Two doors are ajar...

The sadness and sorrow of killing
the unborn is real. Our voice
comes tenderly to you with reason.
We pray that you'll make the right choice.

*What greater gift could you offer
than to let someone living be born?*
How much better it is now to nurture
your child than to let her be torn
into pieces or suctioned or poisoned
by unscrupulous abortionists
who have sterilized, maimed and killed women?
They just want you to feather their nests.

A doctor who delivers live babies
could double his income or more
if he'd stoop to deliver dead babies
and throw bags of them on the floor.

So go to a live baby doctor
 and avoid the abortionist's door!
CHOOSE LIFE! Let your name go on living
 and you'll never be lonely or "poor".

The greatest of "riches" aren't dollars
 or stocks, buildings, silver or gold.
The greatest of "riches" are children...born of
 you...kids to have and to hold!

The wheel of life turns so swiftly.
The brief months of pregnancy pass.
But for those who destroy their own children
 remorse, tears and sorrows amass.

So resolve as you contemplate killing
 that you'll never take that way out.
Then someday someone who needs you
 will run joyfully to you and shout,
"MOMMY! DADDY! GRANDMA! GRANDPA!
 THANKS FOR LOVING ME!!"

"Grandchildren are the crown of the aged,
 and the glory of children is their fathers" (Proverbs 17:6).

"A good man leaves an inheritance to his children's children,
 but the sinner's wealth is laid up for the righteous"
 (Proverbs 13:22).

Even if you have given a child up for adoption, you may love
that child by including him or her in your will.

SOUL CELEBRATION

Soul celebration! Growing strong.
Just beneath your heart there lies a song.
Words unsung. Tongue still forming
   in God's image...heart conforming
   to his mom's...with love awaiting.
You're a'blooming...hesitating.
Can you stand the looks of others?
Some snobs detest unwed mothers.
Some folks think that timing's prime.
They say, "Wait! Another time
   would be better to give birth."
Let those losers watch your girth.
Feed your body the best foods.
Walk the meadows. Bike the woods.
Swim the lakes. And watch your looks.
Start collecting picture books.
Time goes forward. Life exists.
Don't let misdirected twists
   turn you from birthing a soul.
Eternal life needs to be whole.
Don't stop your child from a chance
   to hug and kiss you...and to dance.
There's a first for everything.
It doesn't matter if a ring
   graces your soft mother's hand.
Be a righteous lady. Land
   in the middle of God's will.
Don't bid your child's heart grow still.
Don't yield to pressures for blood.
Don't duck if the pro-choice mud*
   flies at you and at us all.
God used clay to form a man.
Be like God. Create again.
Do your part and you will see
   things work out. Be you. Be free.
Tears of happiness arrive
   when your child is born alive.
Tears of remorse follow her
   who submits to death's detour.

Take the right road. Risk the strife.
Be brave. Be Bold. And hold to life!
Grasp your child, still in your womb.
Be a mom and not a tomb!
Love and be loved. Time will prove
        you chose rightly, chose to love.
There's no doubt there is a soul
        safe inside you. Be peace. Be whole.
Things will work out. Wait and see.
God turns defeat to victory.
Those who've had abortions feel jealousy.
Be you. Be real. Be a mom.

Soul celebration! Growing strong.
Just beneath your heart there lies a song.
Words unsung. Tongue still forming
        In God's image…heart conforming
        to his mom's. He'll model you.
You'll co-create a love that's new.
Each day we face important choices.
Dream a moment. Hear the voices.
"Mommy, Mommy! Look at me!
I can climb an apple tree!"
Children singing. Sunday morn'.
Proud mom's smiling. Hope is born.
"Jesus loves me. This I know.
"Cause my mommy tells me so."
Soul celebration! Growing strong.
Just beneath your heart there lies a song.
Mom, let that song be heard!

*He or she who throws mud loses ground.

YOUR LIFTING LOVE

Lord, I long to embrace all
    You have in store for me.
Sever all the cords that bind me.
Master, set me free!

Let my spirit soar through
    heaven on the wings
    that a sultry summer updraft
    sometimes brings.

Sometimes I feel like a gliding
    sail plane, Lord,
    totally dependent on
    updrafts that soared
    long before I was a twinkle
    in dad's eye.

Precious Holy Spirit,
    do not pass me by.
I can only keep aloft
    if You are here,
    lifting me up from the earth
    and pain and fear.

**Jesus, be the power for
    my every move.
May I rest securely on
    Your lifting love.**

May every gift God's given you
    mature and grow and flower.
May fragrances of His best will
    surround you in this hour.

JUST A SALARIED GUARD

I am just a salaried guard,
　　standing by the door.
The city pays me to keep peace.
Those picketers abhor
　　what is going on inside.
They claim that kids are killed!

I see the pain on faces of
　　the people who work here.
Too often and too loud they joke.
I sense somehow they fear
　　analyzing what they do.

The new girl went out back
　　and lost her lunch, then flew
　　to her car. She laid a strip
　　of rubber on the drive.
She screamed, "The fetus in the trash
　　just wiggled. It's alive!"

She'll never be back. That I know.
　　The turnover is quite high.
Eventually they'll keep their staff.
I see a vulture fly.
That should be the clinic's bird,
　　a mascot on a perch.

God, I hate the job, but I
　　need my check. I lurch
　　as the picketers reach out
　　offering a tract.
I tell them, "Let the clients through!"
I am the prince of tact.

One day a picketer came up.
I thought I knew her face.
She said, "I once came here to have
　　my child killed." The lace
　　on her blouse heaved with anguished pain

and as she wept, she said,
"They told me my problems would end,
    but now my child is dead.
I wouldn't wish abortion on
    anyone else. Their fate
    is better served if I warn them to
    turn back. Don't hesitate."

This very clinic mutilated
    this brave picketer.
I was the guard who walked her through
    that day on death's detour.
**I was once a salaried guard,
    standing by the door...**

PART VII
MEDICAL APPENDIX & TYPES OF ABORTION

Induced abortion is the deliberate termination of a human pregnancy with outside intervention. Spontaneous abortion happens without human intervention. It is commonly referred to as miscarriage.

A CHEMICAL OR MEDICAL ABORTION DOES NOT INVOLVE INSTRUMENTS

(These terms are interchangeable. Both are nonsurgical procedures.)

The Pharmacists for Life organization estimates that **there have been approximately 250 million babies aborted chemically in the United States since 1973!** (http://www. pfli.org/). This is a superb website which also describes other unpublicized things such as illegally selling baby parts. Abortion methods are normally categorized by the age of gestation, that is, how long the woman has been pregnant.

THE MORNING AFTER PILL

This medication is sometimes recommended if a woman has been raped or had unprotected sex.

Levonorgestrel® is a hormone that can be used for emergency contraception. Emergency contraception should not be used as a routine method of birth control.

Levonorgestrel can usually prevent pregnancy after unprotected sex. People sometimes call it THE MORNING AFTER PILL." But you don't have to wait until the morning after sex to take it. In fact, **Levonorgestrel is more effective the sooner you take it after having unprotected sex**. It is a one-dose regimen: you take one pill. The pill contains 1.5 milligrams of Levonorgestrel, which is used in lower doses in many birth control pills.

Levonorgestrel brands include Econtra EZ®, My Way®, Next Choice One Dose®, Plan B One Step®, Preventeza®, and Take Action®. How Does Levonorgestrel Work? Depending upon where you are in your cycle, Levonorgestrel may work in one of these ways:
It may prevent or delay ovulation.
It may interfere with fertilization of an egg.
It is also possible that this type of emergency birth control prevents implantation of a fertilized egg in the uterus by altering its lining.

Levonorgestrel is not the same as RU-486, which is an abortion pill. It does not cause a miscarriage or abortion. In other words, it does not stop development of a fetus once the fertilized egg implants in the uterus. So it will not work if you are already pregnant when you take it.

How effective is Levonorgestrel? If you take it **within 72 hours** after you've had unprotected sex, **Levonorgestrel can reduce the risk of pregnancy by up to 89%.** If you take Plan B One-Step within 24 hours, it is about 95% effective. But you should know that Plan B One-Step is not as effective as regular contraception. So don't take it as your main form of birth control. And, it does not protect you against sexually transmitted diseases. Think of it as a backup -- not for routine use. That's why it's called Plan B. (This information on the morning after pill is from WEBMD: https://www.webmd.com/sex/birth-control/plan-b#1)

CHEMICAL OR NONSURGICAL ABORTION

"Prior to the coronavirus outbreak, **chemical abortion** (https://www.guttmacher.org/evidence-you-can-use/medication-abortion) **already accounted for** (/the-troubling-rise-of-do-it-yourself-abortions) **more than 40% of all U.S. abortions.**" The following procedures can be done in the presence of one's doctor or remotely. These methods are used during the first twelve weeks of pregnancy. An early abortion is most successful when it is done as early as possible after the woman discovers she is pregnant. If the pregnancy test is positive and it has been four weeks since the last period, this means the woman has been pregnant for approximately two weeks. **Early abortions are categorized into medical or nonsurgical abortion and surgical abortion.** If a woman has been pregnant up to seven weeks, this method of medical abortion is 98% effective (https://www.glamcheck. com/health/2011/29/early-abortion). The woman will have to go in for a follow-up appointment and be given a blood test or ultrasound to learn if the early abortion pill has worked. If it has not, a surgical abortion will be needed. It is not uncommon if the woman has learned she is still pregnant, that she decides to continue carrying her baby.

There are conflicting reports about what percentage of mothers having a medical abortion experience complications. It is between one and seven percent. Glamcheck continues and I quote, "More than 99% of the women undergoing early abortion have no adverse side effects or problems…a fraction of the 1% cases result in death… **The following symptoms indicate that something has gone wrong with a mother's abortion: nausea or vomiting more than two days after taking misoprostol in the case of a medical early abortion; high fever that lasts more than 4 to 5 hours; recurring, very large blood clots the size of large lemons; extensive bleeding where the mother is soaking two pads in two hours; smelly vaginal discharge; period like cramps or stomach pain that is very intense and does not go away despite pain medication; resting and other methods of pain management such as using a hot water bottle."**

According to the Food and Drug Administration (FDA) chemical abortions are "designed to induce uterine bleeding and cramping". Beyond those intended effects (https://www. acessdata.fda.gov/drugsatfda_docs/label/2016/020687s020lbl. pdf), numerous women experience weakness, fever/chills, vomiting, diarrhea, dizziness and other complications.

Chemical abortion complications can require surgical follow-up procedures (https://www.ncbi.nlm.nih.gov/pubmed/19888037) or emergency room care in five to seven percent of women.

Complications of chemical abortion (https://www.frc.org/ get.cfm?i=PV19E03) includes ruptured ectopic pregnancies, severe hemorrhaging, infection, and retained pregnancy tissue. *The rates for complications resulting from chemical abortions are four times higher than for a surgical procedure.*

This procedure involves taking two pills. The first is called Mifiprestone (RU-486)®. (The contents of the first pill may also be given as a shot.) This is sometimes given at a family planning clinic or hospital. The woman is sent home after taking this progesterone-inhibitor. A pregnancy needs a hormone called Progesterone 24/7 to continue. Without Progesterone the lining of the wall of the uterus will break down. Because the embryo is attached to the wall, when this happens the pregnancy is terminated. The woman may experience bleeding or spotting when this happens.

The second pill is called Misoprostol®. It is taken 48-72 hours after the first. The woman's doctor will tell her exactly when to take it. This pill will cause uterine cramping and will expel the contents of the uterus. The pain is similar to the cramping a woman experiences during her period. The intensity of the pain may vary from woman to woman. Over-the-counter medication is prescribed to help her manage the discomfort. A woman should not take just any pain medication, as it may have adverse side effects such as excessive bleeding. The bleeding may involve clotting. The clotting is how the woman's body ejects the pregnancy. The bleeding or clotting may last up to a month. No one can predict exactly how long it will continue. Therefore the woman is advised to use sanitary pads rather than tampons during this time.

18 YEAR OLD CHEMICAL ABORTION VICTIM

Monty Patterson testified before the U.S. Subcommittee on Criminal Justice, Drug Policy and Human Resources of the Committee on Government Reform in May of 2006.

"Twelve days after his daughter Holly's 18th birthday on

September 10, 2003, she walked into a Planned Parenthood clinic to be administered an RU-486 medical abortion regimen," her father Monty Patterson said.

"By the fourth day she was admitted to the emergency room of a local hospital," he said. "She was examined. She was given painkillers. She complained of bleeding, cramping, constipation and pain. But subsequently she was sent home."

Seven days after taking RU-486, Holly would return to the same hospital emergency room complaining of weakness, vomiting, abdominal pain, Patterson said.

"Hours later I was called to the hospital where I found her surrounded by doctors and nurses, barely conscious and struggling to breathe," he said.

"Holly was so weak she could barely hold onto my hand," said Monty Patterson. "Feeling utter disbelief and desperation, I watched Holly succumb to a massive bacterial infection as a result of a drug-induced abortion with RU-486."

Patterson detailed how he spent thousands of hours researching medical and scientific journals, talking to doctors, legislators, state and federal agencies, to learn about the drug RU-486.

Chemical abortion, or RU-486, also known as Mifeprex or Mifepristone, is a two-pill process. The first pill stops the mother's womb from building up Progesterone, the necessary hormone for a pregnancy to thrive. The second pill, taken one to two days later, causes the uterus to contract and deliver the deceased fetus.

Chemical abortions, also known as medical or medication abortions, are on the rise and poised to outnumber surgical abortions, now accounting for 40% of all abortions performed in the U.S. The abortion lobby has pushed for greater access to the abortion pill for some time and used the coronavirus pandemic to press for less regulation of the drugs.

"Yet does the average patient, a teenager like Holly, understand she may be risking her life taking RU-486," he continued, "when she's repeatedly exposed to statements like, "It's what women have wanted for years," "It's the first FDA-approved pill, providing women with a safe and active non-surgical option for ending early pregnancy"?"

As of the end of 2018, there had been 24 reported deaths of women in the United States associated with abortion pills. The FDA has also documented at least 4,000 cases of serious adverse events related to the abortion pill, including more than 1,000 women who required hospitalization.

While chemical abortion was being pushed via webcam in the state of Iowa, Iowans for LIFE's Board President Tom Quiner had written an essay about the issue in the Des Moines Register, which prompted Monty Patterson to write him about the risks.

"Medical abortion can be a very dangerous procedure," he told Iowans for Life's board president, Quiner in 2013. "I know firsthand, I held Holly's hand as she fought for her life but eventually succumbed to a horrible and painful death."

"My concern is not about the abortion debate but women's health," Patterson had said.

SUMMARIZE NEGATIVE SIDE EFFECTS OF THE ABORTION PILL

High blood pressure, overgrowth of the uterine lining, low energy, fluid retention in the legs, feet, arms or hands, loss of appetite, head pain, nausea, vomiting, diarrhea, uterine cramps, bleeding not related to menstrual period, low amounts of potassium in the blood, indigestion, inflammation or infection of the vagina, chronic trouble sleeping, fever, chills and dizziness.

ABORTION PILL REVERSAL – AMERICAN PREGNANCY ASSOCIATION

The abortion pill reversal (APR) procedure can only occur after the first dose of medical abortion Mifepristone (RU-486) is taken orally. It is ineffective after the second set of pills Misoprostol is taken. But just as abortion in itself is a controversial topic, so is the idea of being able to reverse a medical abortion. The abortion pill reversal process involves adding a large influx of progesterone into the pregnant woman's system. This is due to the fact that the first pill, Mifepristone, blocks progesterone from being absorbed by the womb. Mifepristone blocks where progesterone would normally be absorbed, so an influx of progesterone can outcompete for the available binding spaces. Some say that treatment with progesterone after the first pill (Mifepristone) is no more effective than just letting nature take its course, and that excess progesterone can be unsafe. Others show that it is more effective and is indeed safe to use progesterone after Mifepristone. So, what is the truth on the subject? Is there enough research or backing to say what works and is safe? **The American Association of Pro-Life Obstetricians and Gynecologists (AAPLOG) believes that the procedure is safe and significantly more effective than "seeing what happens" without the second medication, Misoprostol. The American Pregnancy Association (APA) reports that 64-68% of women who take the abortion pill reversal have seen that their babies are saved.** (24/7/365 helpline for Heartbeat International is 800-712-HELP. They can also direct you where to go to get a free pregnancy test.)

Some pro-choice advocates protest the use of the abortion reversal pill claiming it is a new unproven drug. Danielle White, general counsel for Heartbeat International, denounced this idea and affirmed the APR treatment and its benefit to women, stating, "Contrary to the Campaign for Accountability's surprising assertion, progesterone is not a 'new drug'. Progesterone is a hormone necessary for a healthy pregnancy, and it has been used since the 1950's to prevent threatened miscarriages. **No woman should be forced to complete an unwanted abortion.** Abortion Pill Reversal care gives women a choice to attempt to stop an in-progress abortion – a choice that she should be free to make." I wish to acknowledge Lisa Bourne, the Managing Editor of Pregnancy Help News and Content Writer for Heartbeat International for her excellent research about these topics.

SUGGESTED QUESTIONS TO DISCUSS WITH THE PHYSICIAN OR PERSON WHO WANTS TO ABORT YOUR CHILD

According to the Planned Parenthood website under abortion they assure everyone, "There are two ways of ending a pregnancy: in-clinic abortion and the abortion pill. Both are safe and very common. If you're pregnant and thinking about abortion, you may have lots of questions. We're here to help." (Just because an abortion facility claims that it is safe doesn't make it true. They haven't convinced me that this is true. I will give Planned Parenthood credit for noting that these procedures are "very common".)

In 2019 Planned Parenthood received $616.8 million in government health services reimbursements and grants. They provided 2.4 million people with various services including abortions. **I applaud the additional services which Planned Parenthood provides to support women's overall health** and will soon recommend how they can further serve their clients. That comes out to $257 per person. Other abortion providers also received government funding. I propose that the same amount of money per person helped be distributed to pro-life organizations. List the good or bad things which pro-choice counselors do for our country. Compare that to the good or bad things that pro-life counselors do for our country. Perhaps there should be two tiers for Social Security benefits, one for pro-choice and the other for pro-life tax payers. If it is discovered that pro-life people have larger families, wouldn't it be fair if pro-life parents received larger monthly retirement benefits from Social Security?

Please refer to the inside back cover of this book for

suggested questions you may discuss with the doctor who proposes to sell you an abortion.

I am in favor of having any complications during any abortion reported in detail to the authorities in each state and having this information publicized on the web site of each physician and pro-choice agency. At this time, I understand that abortionists are given the choice to report complications. Not surprisingly, few do. It makes sense for the complications to be reported. Then protocols can be developed to avoid them.

Some of the risks involved with an early abortion might occur if the patient has a pre-existing health condition. It is important that the woman truthfully and accurately gives her doctor her health history. The woman might have an adverse reaction to the abortion medications. Since the pills used in a medical abortion might not work, the woman might have to also undergo a surgical abortion. The woman might be more likely to have uterine or cervical infections. This is why those having an early abortion are frequently given antibiotics.

The mother should be given a hot-line number after her early abortion which she can call 24/7. If she is not entirely convinced the nurse on the other end has satisfied her concerns she has the right to insist on consulting with a physician. 1 to 7% of women who have a chemical abortion experience complications. **(Some of you my readers may enjoy international travel. May I ask, if an airline had a record of 1 to 7% of their flights having severe mechanical problems or crashing, would you still buy a ticket?)**

ECTOPIC OR TUBAL PREGNANCY

The only fool proof way a doctor can always tell if the mother has an ectopic or tubal pregnancy is to give her an ultrasound. In some instances, a woman was tested and found to be pregnant. So she had the contents of her womb aborted, but not examined. (This failure to examine the contents of her womb which were aborted is most likely to occur early in a pregnancy.) Unfortunately in some cases the woman had an undiagnosed tubal pregnancy. In such an instance, eventually the pain from the tubal pregnancy will cause the woman to return to the abortionist and have the malpractice corrected. This is an unacceptable error. The earlier a tubal pregnancy is diagnosed and removed, the safer it is for the mother. You might ask **why it is some abortionists skip having an ultrasound. One of the main reasons is that when a woman sees her live child on the ultrasound, and hears her baby's heartbeat, most change their minds and cancel the abortion, denying the abortionist their fee.** This information is given by Focus on the Family, an organization whose members helped to donate ultrasound devices to many crisis pregnancy clinics. They report over 50% of the women in crisis pregnancies who see a sonogram (also called ultrasound) of their child and hear the baby's heartbeat continue their pregnancy. These ultrasound machines are responsible for helping an estimated 470,000 pregnant women decide to have their babies. (When my personal attorney was expecting his first grandchild, his daughter gave him and his wife who was a judge, a framed photo of the sonogram. They kept it proudly on their grand piano in the living room.)

Abortion causes scars and always damages the walls of the womb. One of the most dangerous places that the scarring can occur is where the fallopian tubes enter the womb. In a normal pregnancy, the woman ovulates and while the egg is passing down the fallopian tube towards the womb, the father's sperm swims to and impregnates the egg. The father's sperm is very small. Even if there is partial scarring over the place the fallopian tube enters the womb, the father's sperm is frequently still able to swim into the fallopian tube and fertilize the mother's egg. As the fertilized egg grows in some cases, it is too big to leave the fallopian tube and enter the mother's womb. This is called an ectopic or tubal pregnancy. It can be life threatening and will require major surgery which can incapacitate one of the mother's two fallopian tubes. The recovery period from this surgery can take six to eight weeks. Once a woman is diagnosed with an ectopic pregnancy, it should be safely removed as soon as possible.

Has there been an increase in ectopic pregnancies in the U.S. since abortion was legalized in 1973?

In 1970 the incidence was 4.8 per 1,000 births. By 1980 it was 14.5 per 1,000 births. (Dept of H.H.S., Morbidity & Morality Weekly Report, Vol. 33, no.15, April 20, 1984) (ABORTION QUESTIONS AND ANSWERS by Dr. & Mrs. J.C. Willke p.104)

Feb 15, 2000: Based on hospital discharge data, the incidence of ectopic pregnancy has risen from 4.5 cases per 1,000 pregnancies in 1970, to 19.7 cases per 1,000 pregnancies in North America and is a leading cause of maternal mortality in the first trimester {American Family Physician, Feb 15, 2000; 61(4):1080-1088, Josie L. Tenore, M.D., S.M., Northwestern University Medical School, Chicago, Illinois}.

(We have started to review the statistics. It is important that you continue to form your opinion about the claims the abortionists make that "abortion is safe".)

The thin walled fallopian tube cannot support this life and it soon ruptures, causing internal bleeding and requiring emergency surgery. Sometimes these women die. (In the US, there were 437 deaths from ruptured fallopian tubes in the past nine years. Medical Tribune, Jan. 26, 1983). Nine of these deaths were after induced abortions. The mothers had their wombs emptied by abortion when, in reality, the tiny baby was lodged in the fallopian tube. Later the tube ruptured and the women died." (Note: evidently these mothers were not given an ultrasound which would have located exactly where the unborn child was growing. **The only foolproof way a pregnant woman can learn if she has an ectopic pregnancy is if she has a sonogram**. Therefore I propose that all pregnant women (1) be given and shown a sonogram, (2) be given an frameable copy of it, (3) be required to listen to her unborn child's heart beat, and (4) sign a form indicating she has done so. Doctors failing to provide these four items should have their medical license suspended for nine months and be required to pay the mother $5,000. Violations will be posted on their web page.

TYPES OF SURGICAL ABORTION

A surgical abortion uses instruments such as a vacuum device, a syringe or spoon shaped instrument with a sharp edge called a curet. Also needed is a pointed hollow metal tube called a trochar which is hooked up to the vacuum. Besides metal rods of increasing diameter which are used to open up the cervix, abortionists sometimes use lamanari sticks. They are made out of kelp, a type of seaweed which when placed in the vagina absorbs moisture and opens it up so the abortionist can access the unborn child. By searching the internet for the names of these various "instruments of abortion", you may view them.

VACUUM ASPIRATION IS ALSO CALLED SUCTION CURETTAGE, DILATION AND CURETTAGE OR D&C

The method most doctors favor from seven to twelve weeks is vacuum aspiration. The child is attached to the wall of the uterus with a placenta. The umbilical cord transfers the nutrients from the placenta to the child's stomach. The doctor inserts a thin suction tube and/or a looped shaped knife to separate the placenta from the wall of the uterus. Then the doctor vacuums out the uterine lining, embedded placenta and growing child. **As the child grows older, and approaches 12 weeks of age, the child may be dismembered or cut into smaller pieces so that he or she might be suctioned out of his or her mother's womb.** The procedure takes five to ten minutes.

DILATION AND EVACUATION or D&E – SOME MEDICAL PROFESSIONALS PRIVATELY CALL IT DISMEMBERMENT AND EVACUATION

This is the most common abortion technique for second and third trimester abortions. It is generally done when a mother's child is from 12-28 weeks old. It involves the doctor forcibly opening (or dilating) the cervix (the bottom part of the uterus connected to the vagina or birth canal). Then the uterus is scraped and the unborn child and placenta are taken out in pieces. If the unborn child is older other instruments are used to remove the baby. The opening to the womb is enlarged by inserting instruments of increasingly large diameter into the birth canal. It is while forcing these instruments into the womb that the pressure the abortionist uses can accidently cause the tool to enter the womb suddenly and keep going so that it penetrates the wall of the uterus.

SALINE ABORTIONS

In a normal pregnancy, the unborn child is floating and growing in embryonic fluid which is contained within the protective barrier called an embryonic sac. Saline abortions are performed from the 12th through the 28th week of pregnancy. When a child is eleven weeks old, the child begins breathing the amniotic fluid. This type of abortion involves a long needle being inserted through the mother's abdomen into the baby's amniotic fluid. Some of the fluid is drawn out. It is replaced with the abortion fluid. The poison kills the baby by attacking the respiratory system and by burning the skin. Later, the mother delivers a dead or dying baby. The color of the aborted baby may be scalded red.

Once when a doctor was performing a saline abortion without using an ultrasound, the poisonous liquid was accidentally injected into the mother instead of the embryonic sac. Unfortunately the mother died. **I propose legislation mandating that saline abortions may only be done if they include the use of an ultrasound before and during the procedure.**

PROTECTING THE UNBORN CHILD FROM PAIN – ARE ABORTIONISTS WORSE THAN HITLER?

The least an abortionist should be able to do is to make certain a child being aborted is given something to block the pain. Please remember that during an abortion the heartbeat of a child speeds up 300% faster than before the procedure. At least when Hitler was killing Jews during WWII, most of them were gassed. Neonatologist Robin Pierucci has viewed prematurely born infants at the age of viability where they could survive living outside the womb, 24 weeks. This doctor noted how they reacted to painful procedures. "For example when you poke them for blood work…they wrinkle their face… or smack at the offending person." Her research was reported as part of an insider's view on the science behind "The Pain-Capable Unborn Child Protection Act on January 29, 2018."

In 2016 the Journal of Pain Research concluded that "an early form of pain may appear from the 15th week of gestation onward." I found these quotations on the internet when I asked, "How old does a child in the womb have to be to feel pain during an abortion?"

(On a personal note, my best friend lived next door to our family when we were in fourth, fifth and sixth grades. We were 44 and they were 40 Canterbury Court in Teaneck, NJ. My classmate Freddy Wiesenbeck's parents Curt and Miriam were German Jews who escaped from Hitler by riding their bicycles over the Alps. At one point while going downhill, Miriam told me the brakes on her bike failed and she had to dump her bike. She was hurt, and her bike was damaged, but Curt repaired it and they rode on to safety. Miriam told me about how Hitler smashed the hands of a famous Jewish violinist, destroying his ability to perform. How cruel. But ask any abortionist this, "Was what Hitler did as despicable as someone who literally takes a forceps and pulls the arms and legs off an infant growing beneath his mother's heart?" When Miriam got pregnant again, she complained to my mother that she prayed she would have a girl, because Freddy and his younger brother Tommy caused their parents so much trouble. She said, "If it is a boy I would rather that he die." Unfortunately during the child's birth, the umbilical cord wound around his throat killing him. Miriam deeply regretted her prayer and mom comforted her. I added this story to encourage you to be careful about how you pray if you are having a crisis pregnancy.)

PROSTAGLANDIN
This is a hormone-like compound injected into the uterus to cause premature labor. The baby is usually born too early to survive, but live births are possible.

INTRACARDIAC INJECTION
In Intracardiac Injection, the chemical digoxin is injected into the baby's heart. The chemical is designed to cause immediate death. Sometimes these chemicals are injected into the umbilical cord. **The purpose of these chemicals is to stop the baby's heart. They do not always work, so the child is born alive. Live birth is called a "complication of**

abortion." Mothers should ask their abortionist if they have a late term abortion what they would do if this happened to their baby. Different states have different laws about the options the attending physician may take when this happens.

PARTIAL BIRTH ABORTION – THE WORLD'S MOST IMMORAL SURGERY

This procedure is allowed in some states. **The best definition of partial birth abortion that I have found so far is this one which follows from National Right to Life.** I urge you to search the internet for "What is partial birth abortion?" Please view the photos and learn more about it.

What is Partial-Birth Abortion?

Partial-Birth Abortion is a procedure in which the abortionist pulls a **living baby** feet-first out of the womb and into the birth canal (vagina), except for the head, which the abortionist purposely keeps lodged just inside the cervix (the opening to the womb). The abortionist punctures the base of the baby's skull with a surgical instrument, such as a long surgical scissors. He then inserts a catheter (tube) into the incision, and removes the baby's brain with a powerful suction machine. This usually causes the skull to collapse, after which the abortionist completes the delivery of the now-dead baby. If the baby's skull does not collapse when the vacuum removes the brain, the abortionist may crush it with his forceps. Sometimes the splinters from the baby's skull can harm the uterus.

What is the Partial-Birth Abortion Ban Act?

The ***Partial-Birth Abortion Ban Act*** would ban performance of a partial-birth abortion except if it were necessary to the save a mother's life. The bill defines partial-birth abortion as an abortion in which "the person performing the abortion deliberately and intentionally vaginally delivers a living fetus until, in the case of a head-first presentation, the entire fetal head is outside the body of the mother, or, in the case of breech presentation, any part of the fetal trunk past the navel is outside the body of the mother," and then kills the baby. The bill would only permit use of the procedure if "necessary to save the life of a mother whose life is endangered by a physical disorder, physical illness, or physical injury, including a life-endangering physical condition caused by or arising from the abortion."

Are Partial-Birth Abortions Common?

According to Ron Fitzsimmons, executive director of the National Coalition of Abortion Providers (1997), and other sources, it appears that partial-birth abortions are performed 3,000 to 5,000 times annually. (Even those numbers may be low.) Based on published interviews with numerous abortionists and interviews with Fitzsimmons in 1997, the "**vast majority**" of partial-birth abortions are performed in the fifth and sixth months of pregnancy, **on healthy babies of healthy mothers**.

Why is it called "Partial-Birth"?

Under state laws, a "live birth" occurs when a baby is entirely expelled from the mother and shows any signs of life, however briefly -- regardless of whether the baby is "viable," i.e. developed enough to be sustained outside the womb with neo-natal medical assistance. Although at 20 weeks, perinatologists say that if a baby is expelled or removed completely from the uterus, he or she will usually gasp for breath and sometimes survive for hours, even though lung development is usually insufficient to permit successful sustained respiration until 23 weeks. (However 20 week old infants have survived.) Thus, the term "partial-birth abortion" is perfectly descriptive.

I don't know how a mother can instruct her abortionist to do these procedures. I just conclude by saying I believe it is wrong. Your thoughts?

Another valuable resource regarding Abortion Risks is the Louisiana and Texas Department of State Health Services. Another prime source of much of this information is Rama International. I am indebted to all my resources.

A DEVELOPING HUMAN BABY

DAY 1: conception: all 46 human chromosomes present; a unique human life begins.

DAYS 3-4: the father's sperm enters the mother's egg and the fertilized egg travels down the fallopian tube into the womb.

DAYS 5-9: fertilized egg implants itself into the rich lining of the uterus and begins to draw nourishment.

DAY 18: heart begins to beat with blood often of a different type than the mother's blood type.

DAY 30: embryo is 10,000 times larger than the original fertilized egg.

WEEK 5: eyes, hands, feet begin to develop.

WEEK 6: brain waves detectable; mouth, lips present.

WEEK 7: eyelids, fingers and toes form, nose is distinct, and eggs begin to be formed in the unborn girl's body.

WEEK 8: all body systems are present; bones and the nervous system which enables the child to sense pain begin to be formed. By the end of the second month, the baby is about 1 inch long and weighs about 1/30th of an ounce. If we tickle the baby's lips, he will flex his head backward away from the stimulus.

WEEK 9: fingernails develop; baby can suck his or her thumb, kick, curl toes, and bend fingers.

WEEK 10: the embryo is now a fetus. If you stroke the palm, the baby makes a fist.

WEEK 11: baby can smile, begins to breathe amniotic fluid.

MONTH 3: circulatory and urinary systems are working and the liver produces bile. The baby is about 4 inches long and weighs about 1 ounce.

MONTH 4: baby can have dream (REM) sleep, ears are functioning and can hear parents' voices, umbilical cord transports 300 quarts of fluid per day. **One father regularly read the Bible to his unborn son.** Minutes after his son was born, the infant went into distress. Fortunately at that moment, **when the father who was in the delivery room spoke calmly to his infant son, his son recognized his voice and immediately calmed down.** Since the baby's most critical development has taken place, the chance of miscarriage drops considerably after three months. **Most mothers feel movement between weeks 16 to 18.**

MONTH 5: Dr. & Mrs. J. C. Willke in his book ABORTIONS, QUESTIONS AND ANSWERS on p.60 reports, "Marcus Richards was born at 19 weeks 6 days on January 1, 1972 at Cincinnati's University Hospital. He weighed 780 grams" (27.5 ounces). "Melissa Comer was born at 20 weeks on December 1983 at Sault Ste. Marie Hospital in Cincinnati. She weighed only 450 grams" (15.9 ounces). (I saw a pre-school aged child who weighed 16 ounces at birth at a pro-life event in Minneapolis who was enjoying riding his tricycle. Enroute to reversing Roe vs. Wade I would personally endorse prohibiting abortions later than the age of the youngest child who survived a premature birth.) A loud noise may cause the child to jump in the womb in reaction to the sound. Prenatal baby bump shows.

MONTH 6: by the end of the sixth month, your baby is about 12 inches long and weighs about 2 pounds. During the sixth month of her relative Elizabeth's pregnancy…God sent the angel Gabriel to give a message to the Virgin Mary that she would be visited by the Holy Spirit and bare a child who would be the Son of God. Soon after conceiving Mary visited Elizabeth. When Elizabeth heard Mary's greeting, Elizabeth told Mary *""As soon as I heard your greeting the baby within me jumped with gladness"* (Luke 1:41**). In this gospel, the author and physician Luke reports interfetal communication.** Elizabeth's six month old child sensed Mary's recently conceived child. Study the chapter. An unborn child can influence people for good even while he or she is spending time in the mother's womb. The chapter documents how two Godly pregnant women celebrated the gift of the lives they were carrying.

MONTH 7: at the end of the seventh month, the baby is about 14 inches long and weighs from 2 to 4 pounds. The baby uses the four senses of vision, hearing, taste and touch. He or she changes position frequently and responds to stimuli, including sound, pain, and light. The amniotic fluid begins to diminish.

MONTH 8: the baby is about 18 inches long and weighs as much as 5 pounds. The skin begins to thicken with a layer of fat stored underneath it for insulation and nourishment, antibodies are increasingly built up, amniotic fluid is completely replaced every three hours.

MONTH 9: 90% of babies are born between 266 and 294 days from the first day after the mother's last menstrual period, infants normally weigh 6 to 9 pounds. The baby's heart is pumping 250 gallons of blood per day and he or she is fully capable of surviving outside of the womb. The baby's reflexes are coordinated. The baby is definitely ready to enter the world.

Sources: Focus on the Family, "THE FIRST NINE MONTHS." For a brochure or to discuss your pregnancy with a trained counselor at no cost, call 1-800-AFAMILY. See also Cleveland Clinic: https://my.clevelandclinic.org/health/articles/7247-fetal-development-stages-of-growth

PHYSICAL DAMAGE -
THE MYTH OF A SAFE ABORTION

Has any pro-choice advocate ever proven that there is such a thing as a "safe abortion"? **Before you get an abortion, insist on being shown statistical proof that they are telling you the truth.** *Show them for example the statistics on breast cancer in this book. Challenge them to refute our evidence.*

Abortion is never safe! The first thing any mother having a crisis pregnancy should remember is that she may be aborting the only child she may ever conceive. Any woman who has an abortion has an increased risk of sterility, having a tubal pregnancy, being unable to carry a child to term or having her next child suffering from preventable birth defects.

The uterus is the place where a woman's child grows during pregnancy. The lower third of the uterus is called the cervix. It is about two inches long prior to pregnancy. A healthy cervix insures the mother's womb can safely hold her growing child for a full nine month term. But in order to remove the unborn child from the womb, the abortionist foolishly and forcibly permanently stretches the cervix. The painful unnecessary damage can never be fully reversed.

Abortion results in cervical damage, which causes a permanent weakening of the cervix, which, in turn, may be unable to carry the weight of a later pregnancy. The injured cervix opens prematurely. A survey by Dr. Ren, "Cervical Incompetence - Aetiology and Management," Medical Journal of Australia, December 29, 1993, Volume 60, reported that **"symptoms related to cervical incompetence were found among 75% of women who undergo forced dilation for abortion."**

WHY RISK ABORTING THE ONLY CHILD YOU WILL EVER CONCEIVE?

"The risk of secondary infertility among women with at least one induced abortion is 3-4 times greater than that among non-aborted women." (British Journal of OB/GYN, August, 1976)

Dr. Bohumil Stipal, Czechoslovakia's Deputy Minister of Health, stated, **"Roughly 25% of the women who interrupt their first pregnancy have remained permanently childless."** Is it significant to you that if you have an abortion the odds are one in four that you may never conceive another child?

When a mother has an abortion the procedure by which the vaginal canal is forcibly dilated and the unborn child is scraped from the wall of her womb, could cause permanent scarring. Some abortions involve inserting poison into the amniotic fluid, the umbilical cord or the heart of the unborn child. This procedure can also damage the wall of the mother's womb. **Because the fluid is strong enough to burn the infant to death, imagine the damage it does to the walls of the mother's womb.** The placenta needs a healthy wall of the mother's womb in order to attach normally and give the right mixture of nutrients to the mother's next child. **(I read a comment about a woman who urged other women to have an abortion. She bragged that she had had one and later birthed a healthy child. She did not realize that if the inside of her womb had scars, then her child might have had a lower IQ or hidden injuries** because damage to her womb prevented her child from getting the ideal amount of nutrients.) Ask yourself, **"Do I want the next child I conceive to have the optimum mixture of nutrients throughout the whole nine months of a full term pregnancy?"** Don't just mentally consider this thought. Write the question down and **meditate on it daily until you decide if you wish to let an abortionist end the life of your unborn child.** The child beneath your heart as you read this paragraph deserves a healthy sibling, one with normal intelligence, one who is physically fit, and in superb health, one with an unmutilated mother, a mother with enlarged shapely healthy natural feminine breasts who has no inhibitions about being romantic with her man. Such a mother can live and make love with her husband joyously without guilt. She loves and is loved by the child she is carrying, and all her future children.

Let's suppose you enter an abortion facility and are talking to a woman on staff there to decide whether or not you should have an abortion. Why not ask the woman with whom you are talking, "Have you had an abortion experience? Did you have any complications or reservations?" Let the woman with whom you are talking share from her heart. Do not rush past these discussion points.

(The ideas in this present paragraph are obviously optional. Don't feel obligated to share them. But let's suppose you are pregnant and talking about these things with a woman for example working in an abortion facility who admitted she had had an abortion and that sometimes she has been jealous of a mother who had a healthy infant, you might ask, "May I give you a hug?" *It is ok to comfort your counselor.* If you are unsure whether or not you should have an abortion, tell her so. Then ask, "Would you like to resign right now and walk out of this place with me?")

A certain fisherman caught a massive salmon when he was fishing on a river in Oregon. It was so big, he took a lot of pictures of it, weighed it, then cleaned and ate it. A few days later, he found out it was a world record. But he couldn't get credit for catching it because he didn't recognize how unique and special it was and bring it to the authorities to be certified. As you consider the future you want for your unborn child, do not doubt that your child is unique, special and has enormous potential to bless you, your family and perhaps the world. Don't be like the fisherman who failed to see the uniqueness in that exceptional salmon.

Keep in mind that a major goal of an abortionist is to do as many procedures in as short a time as possible. Those of you who have attended the birth of a child will recall the nurse keeps track of how many centimeters her birth canal is dilated. In a normal birth God designed the birth canal to open gradually and safely so that every child can be delivered at full term into the waiting arms of his or her loving parents. But abortionists want to force the womb open so they can swiftly reach in and remove the child and placenta from the mother's womb.

In a normal birth of her first born child, labor may last 24 or more hours. During this time, the opening to the womb slowly and naturally relaxes and enlarges. By contrast, an abortionist may force it to open in only a couple of minutes.

I have heard that one movie star had some abortions. Later when she desired to have a child she suffered some miscarriages. In order to safely carry a child to term on the advice of her OB doctor she spent the last few months of her pregnancy in total bed rest. Subsequently she bore a healthy child.

One of the saddest stories I ever heard involved a 23 year old woman who was harmed by an abortionist. It happened when the doctor inserted a suction tube into her womb. He accidentally penetrated the wall of her womb and sucked out a major part of her colon. From that day forward she had to wear an ugly, smelly and inconvenient colostomy bag.

Sometimes the father of the child threatens to unfairly terminate the relationship with the mother unless she has an abortion. The number of weeks before a couple breaks up following an abortion is surprisingly small.

Is there such a thing as an unwanted child? The waiting time most adoption agencies have is so long that many adoption agencies are no longer taking applications because there are not enough children to go around. Even children with birth defects have couples who are willing to give them a loving home. If you learn that the child you are carrying may have a birth defect and you are unsure about raising it, look on the internet to learn if someone might still be willing to adopt your differently-abled child. (See also pages 66, 166, 170 and 193.)

Pro-lifers should not patronize companies that send money to organizations that promote abortion. **Family Council** (https://familycouncil.org/) is a conservative education and research organization that promotes, protects and strengthens traditional family values found and reflected in the Bible. **They maintain a list of the numerous large U.S. corporations that have contributed money directly to Planned Parenthood**. In addition, abortion-rights political and professional organizations such as the Democratic Party, Emily's List, the Feminist Abortion Network, the National Abortion Federation, African-American Women for Reproductive Freedom, American Civil Liberties Union promote and support abortion. **Don't they realize they are reducing the number of workers needed to keep America and social security solvent?**

Instead of donating money to companies like Planned Parenthood who encourage ending the lives of unborn children we urge you to study and invest in the organizations in our enclosed resource list. Japan and Germany are two nations where the ratio of workers to retired people is dangerously low. (Research this on your own.) To compensate for the lack of workers to keep their factories going, Germany has drastically lowered immigration requirements so workers for example from Muslim nations can move there. This policy has created its own set of problems.

I would favor legislation that calculates the ideal number of babies and immigrants the United States needs to have each year in order to have the healthiest economy. We could also do our utmost to hire immigrants of child bearing age with specific needed skills to help boost our economy. Canada wisely gives foreign students the option of citizenship when they finish college. So should America. These new citizens could boost our economy. We frequently send students back to their country of origin when they finish their post high school education. Legislators should focus on welcoming a higher percentage of immigrants with stronger education credentials. The system is set up so people are supposed to be in line in order to be admitted to the United States. It is totally unfair for illegals to cut into the line and enter before those who are following the correct method of immigrating to our country. I am against illegals getting any financial benefit from our government.

BORDER WALL – USER FEES

(I will comment on various current issues.) In addition **I am in favor of building a secure wall across America's southern border.** I believe it should be partially funded by user fees. Vehicles should be charged $2.00 per tire. Persons entering or leaving the United States would be charged $5.00 each time they cross the border. Persons crossing our border by train, bus, plane or boat will also be charged $5.00. Mexico already charges people who enter their country. These fees would also apply to our northern continental border.

ABORTION INCREASES THE ODDS OF THESE THINGS GOING WRONG

Conceiving a child
Having a tubal pregnancy
Having a miscarriage
Delivering a child prematurely
Having the child suffer various birth defects
Having the mother suffer emotionally from post abortion syndrome (PAS)
Having a wide assortment of medical problems such as breast cancer.

Therefore **I think it's only fair that the abortion clinics pick up part of the tab for mothers who suffer these complications.** Furthermore, even as insurance companies have a separate set of rates for smokers, women who have had an abortion should pay more for their health and life insurance. Last I heard, New York doesn't even increase the cost of malpractice insurance for doctors who perform abortions. This means pro-life OB/GYN physicians are unfairly forced to share in the cost of malpractice insurance with pro-choice physicians. After all, abortionists are more likely to have medical and legal expenses than their ethical pro-life counterparts.

Abortionists present themselves as being loving and caring for the welfare of the woman in a crisis pregnancy. So do **pro-life advocates. Which group cares the most?** Which of these two groups charges for their services and which freely donate their time to help women in crisis pregnancies? Which group gives out layettes? *"Blessed is the man whose sin the Lord does not count against him and in whose spirit there is no deceit. When I kept silent, my bones wasted away through my groaning all day long. For day and night your hand was heavy upon me. My strength was dried up as in the heat of summer. Then I acknowledged my sin to you and did not cover up my iniquity. I said, 'I will confess my transgressions to the Lord' and you forgave the guilt of my sin"* (Taken from my favorite Psalm 32:2-5).

Many former abortionists have switched over to the pro-life side. Check out the 1984 film clip "THE SILENT SCREAM". The man who at that time had performed more abortions than anyone in America saw a sonogram of an unborn child in the womb trying to swim away from a wand which being used to suction and end the unborn child's life. (I might note that the quality of the image on an ultrasound had undergone a lot of improvement since 1973 when abortion was legalized.)

The expression on the child's face was a SILENT SCREAM. The child's desire to live caused Dr. Bernard Nathanson to switch to the pro-life camp. (You might want to ask the computer "Which abortionists became pro-life?") While visiting the pro-choice booth at the 2019 Minnesota State Fair, I asked the three women there, "Why does the heartbeat of a child who is being aborted beat 300 percent faster?" They avoided the question, admitted they have different views than pro-life advocates and said we should just accept the fact differences occur. While riding a bus to offsite parking following a visit to the Minnesota State Fair in 2016 I asked the woman sitting next to me what she did for a living. She said she was a social worker who counseled pregnant teenage girls. I said, "Oh great, you are pro-life then?" She said, "Definitely not." I asked her, "When does life begin?" She took offense, raised her voice and said with finality, "I don't want to talk about it. I just came to the fair to have fun." I prayed about what to say next. Not sensing anything, I respected her request and kept silent until she was leaving the bus. Then I said, "Have fun."

There is another complication which can harm the mother who has an abortion. **SOMETIMES NOT ALL OF THE PARTS OF HER BABY AND THE PLACENTA ARE REMOVED DURING THE ABORTION.** What might the abortionist do to reduce the odds of any part of the fetus being left in the womb where they might cause infection? Ideally the parts are assembled when removed. (If the fetus is small, it might be difficult to verify the abortion was complete.) The doctor should offer to show the mother what was taken from her womb and give her photos. Photos should also go into the patient's permanent chart.

We need to be certain abortionists and coroners can never again cover up their mistakes. While researching this book, I recall reading observations by a pathologist who did an autopsy of a woman who died during an abortion. The parts of the death certificate which indicated the cause of death had been blacked out. The person who did the autopsy had specifically attributed the details of this unfortunate mother's death to a medical mistake which the abortionist had made. The conclusion the woman who did the autopsy made was that **the abortion provider was able to influence coroners to keep the physician who did this abortion from being held responsible for this mother's death.** This totally inexcusable illegal hiding of the abortionist's mistake should be prosecuted to the full extent of the law. The abortionist and the person who blacked out that information on the death certificate should be identified and held accountable. **That dead woman's family deserves appropriate compensation.** I ask the person who blotted out this information to come forward and re-instigate the cause of death so that justice can be done.

THE EMOTIONAL SIDE EFFECTS FOLLOWING ABORTION ARE MORE COMMON THAN THE PHYSICAL SIDE EFFECTS

GENERAL DISCUSSION - IS IT WORTH RISKING HAVING THESE SIDE EFFECTS?
Following an abortion some mothers have a preoccupation with babies and getting pregnant again and worry about how close to get to their significant other. Should the relationship go forward or terminate? For sure those who have had an abortion need a safe person with whom they can share what they are experiencing. In order to be the best you can be you need to have your act together. If a woman doesn't have a positive self image, then she risks hindering her academic, professional, personal and interpersonal success. **Suppose a woman decides to keep her child, but later finds out the situation wasn't working. She can still exercise the**

adoption option, whereas if one ends the life of their child, there is no plan B.

Women commonly report that the abortion procedure affected them more than they expected it would. Some individuals are more susceptible to experiencing various types of negative emotional or psychological side effects. They include individuals with previous emotional or psychological concerns, individuals who have been coerced, forced or persuaded to get an abortion (when deep in their heart they would have preferred to love their child and give him or her the chance to live happy, healthy, productive emotional, physical and spiritual lives). Individuals with religious, moral or ethical beliefs that conflict with abortion, individuals who abort in the later stages of pregnancy, individuals without support from significant others or their partner, and individuals obtaining abortion for genetic or fetal abnormalities may experience increased problems.

What might someone who is considering an abortion do? Get help. Avoid isolation. Don't withdraw from others or keep the matter a secret. Especially involve the grandparents. (I remember talking over this type of scenario with my son when he was starting to date. Before our conversation ended, my son knew that in the unlikely situation that he might ever be facing an unplanned pregnancy, I would back him all the way and help him work through the challenges. My son wisely committed to never having an abortion.) In the event of an unplanned pregnancy don't just talk about it with your friends. If you discuss whether or not to abort your child with a woman who has had an abortion, in order to consciously or subconsciously justify her bad decision, she may urge you to kill your child. **Seek the opinion of a qualified counselor who will help you evaluate your options. Write out and carefully study the options and the implications of each. Your counselor can help you identify them. But you must choose for yourself and your child what you will do. If you took the advice of your counselor and it turned out to be good, then you could never take full credit for the decision. On the other hand, if the advice didn't work out, you could blame the counselor for giving you bad advice.**

Avoid pressure. Whether you keep and raise your child or offer your child to a loving qualified family or person, you and your child are going to have to live with your choice. Seek out people who have gone through an unplanned pregnancy and find out what it was like for them. There are volunteers at pro-life counseling clinics eager to talk with you and many will also share their abortion experience. Study the lives of successful people who were adopted. Get to know people who were adopted. See how beautiful the decision their parents made to let them live and experience the joys and challenges of life can be. Finally, get an ultrasound photo and if possible a video of your unborn child. Take it home with you. Show it to your loved ones. Peace awaits. You were made to live, love and make wise best choices.

This next sentence is the biggest understatement in the whole book, *"In my research about the abortion issue, I have come to realize that well paid people involved in the abortion industry cannot be relied upon to always act responsibly or in their clients' best interest."*

POST ABORTION SYNDROME (PAS) – DO YOU WISH TO RISK HAVING THESE EMOTIONAL PROBLEMS?

METICULOUS MEASURED SUMMARY BY EXPERTS
Five factors or criteria identify a woman who is suffering from PAS. First, the woman experiences the stress of the event itself with all the emotional turmoil that goes along with making the decision, having the procedure and interacting with principal people in her life. These may include her marriage partner, lover, parents, counselors, clergy and friends.

Second, the woman re-experiences the event in her memory or by dreaming about the procedure or child. She might feel like the abortion is reoccurring and that she is lying on the surgical table with her feet in the stirrups, feeling the painful forced dilation of her cervix and watching the abortionist take the child out of her body. Let the abortionist offer to position the screen so both he and the mother can see everything. THE AMERICAN PSYCHIATRIC ASSOCIATION confirmed the existence of PAS in 1980. Dr. Vincent M. Rue presented a paper on "Current Status and Trends in the Study of PAS" on July 19, 1987 to the Second National Conference on Post Abortion Counseling at the University of Notre Dame. The emotional and psychological symptoms include, "depression, grief, anxiety, sadness, shame, helplessness, sorrow, lowered self-esteem, distrust, hostility toward self and others, regret, insomnia, recurring dreams, nightmares, anniversary reactions, suicidal behavior, alcohol and/or chemical dependencies, sexual dysfunction, insecurity, numbness, painful re-experiencing of the abortion, relationship disruption, communication impairment, isolation, fetal fantasies, self-condemnation, flashbacks, uncontrollable weeping, eating disorders, preoccupation, distorted thinking, bitterness and a sense of loss and emptiness."

Third, the woman experiences an avoidance phenomenon— that is she becomes less involved with her external world in one or more areas such as a sense of detachment from others, a reduced ability to feel or express emotions, depression, less communication and/or increased hostile interactions. One woman lamented, "I used to grieve for dead babies or hurt children. Now I feel nothing."

Fourth, the woman may experience associated symptoms including hyper alertness, exaggerated startle reaction, explosive hostile outbursts, sleep problems, feeling guilty because she survived when her child did not, the inability to forgive herself for her involvement, memory impairment, trouble concentrating and avoidance of activities which remind her of her abortion.

Fifth, the woman will fall into one of three categories, being stressed, not being stressed, or being likely to become stressed in the future. The same conference at Notre Dame estimated that **from 17-50% of women who have experienced abortions suffer from some degree of PAS**. To you my friends who recognize these symptoms, please get professional counseling and encouragement from your local pro-life clinics, clergy or the post abortion support groups. Use the resource section of this book.

To any couple who goes to an abortion facility, why not ask how if every woman is entitled to a "safe and legal abortion," so many of their clients are surprised when they experience these symptoms? *Get your abortionist to commit in writing that if you let them give you a safe abortion they will totally support you and help you to regain your health.*

I wish to acknowledge three resources for their excellent contributions on these subjects. In CRADLE MY HEART Kim Ketola writes with understanding and an empathetic voice resulting in healing from the trauma of abortion. "In working directly with the pro-life movement over the last few years, I have seen the incredible need for a book such as this one... through powerful real stories, many of them from her own life, Kim graciously communicates the love and hope Jesus brings to hearts wounded by abortion." (Rebecca St. James, singer, author, actress). I also recommend Nancy Michaels for her book, HELPING WOMEN RECOVER FROM ABORTION and Jeanette Vought who wrote POST ABORTION TRAUMA, NINE STEPS TO RECOVERY.

NONHORMONAL BIRTH CONTROL OPTIONS

I suggest you go to this website first:
https://www.webmd.com/sex/birth-control/non-hormonal-birth-control-options
On this website you will learn:
- What is Nonhormonal Birth Control
- Why choose Nonhormonal Birth Control
- Types of Nonhormonal Birth Control (they include the Diaphragm, Cervical Cap, Sponge, Copper IUD, Spermicide, Vaginal Gel, Male Condom, and Female Condom)

There are also Behavioral Methods: Outercourse and the Pull Out Method. (Did you know that sometimes shortly after a man is sterilized he still can conceive a child? This is because he still has sperm in his reproductive organs. Therefore my friends, don't place too much faith in avoiding pregnancy by using the pull out method.)

Natural Family Planning includes: Couple to Couple League, PO Box 111184, Cincinnati, OH 45211 (513) 661-7612. You would do well to request their brochure, "What Does the Catholic Church Really Teach About Birth Control." The two most popular modern methods are the Sympto-Thermal Method and The Ovulation Method. They are a far cry from Calendar Rhythm which was based just on past cycle history.

THE SYMPTO-THERMAL METHOD HAS EFFECTIVENESS
RATES IN THE SAME RANGE AS THE PILL AND THE IUD
AND IS MORE EFFECTIVE THAN THE CONTRACEPTIVE
BARRIER METHODS.
I believe that the most complete book on the subject is THE
ART OF NATURAL FAMILY PLANNING, by John and Sheila
Kippley (Cincinnati: The Couple to Couple League, 1980).

Internet Resources for Natural Family Planning:

ORGANIZATION	WEBSITE
BOMA-USA	http://boma-usa.org
Couple to Couple League	http://cccli.org/
Family of the Americas Foundation	http://www.familyplanning.net
Fertility Awareness Center	http://www.fertaware.com
Georgetown University Institute for Reproductive Health	http://www.irh.org
Justisse Healthworks for Women	http://www.justisse.ca

GREAT REGRETS

A certain teenage boy named his car "Great Regrets". This
way when he took his date back to her home he could tell her,
"I leave you with great regrets."

May I get your opinion of something? "Imagine with me
that there was a woman who had used the pill, but still got
pregnant as 6 to 9% of them do. (17% of the women who
have abortions were taking the pill during the month they
conceived.) She opted to have an abortion. Suppose she
subsequently got breast cancer and had an ugly deforming
mastectomy and had opted not to get implants. If this woman
had an opportunity to bring her unborn child back to life and
have her breasts back not only in their original condition,
but delightfully larger and more attractive, and if she could
hold, love and nurse her child, would she take that option?"
Imagine she had just had her bandages removed after her
mastectomy. She is looking at herself in the mirror through

tears streaming down her face. She is wondering what the man in her life whose love and support she needs now more than ever would think of her. Would she be joyful or have great regrets that she had decided to have the procedure?

Would she go back to her abortionist and thank him or her profusely for giving her a safe abortion? Would she continue to berate pro-life picketers who offered their friendship and help to women entering the abortion facility where her child died? Would she continue her membership in the pro-choice Democratic Party and donate her hard earned money to and only vote for pro-choice political candidates? Would she continue to shop at businesses who donated funds to abortion facilities like Planned Parenthood? (For the poll takers, if 100 percent of women who suffered from breast cancer following their being on the pill had voted pro-life, do you think it would have changed the outcome of the 2020 presidential election? Do you think that 100% of the women who took the pill and who suffered breast cancer were aware of how taking the pill increased the odds of their getting breast cancer? Did pro-life candidates present the arguments against abortion with enough skill and enthusiasm?)

I remember a TV game show called LET'S MAKE A DEAL. The TV emcee had a signature question for the contestants, "DEAL OR NO DEAL?"

Every child in the womb wants to live. Imagine if you will, your child negotiating with you. "Mom, if you agree to love me and give me life, I will agree to love you back and help you keep your breasts. So Mom, 'DEAL OR NO DEAL?' ".

Rather than viewing your unborn child as a problem to be disposed of, why not read the next segment in CHOOSE LIFE and learn how your child is able to prevent you from getting breast cancer?

DANGERS OF THE PILL AND HORMONAL BASED CONTRACEPTION

What medical problems does a woman face when she considers hormonal based contraception? The best site I have ever discovered which discusses these issues is the **Breast Cancer Prevention Institute**. www.bcpinstitute. org. Their founder and president, Dr. Angela Lanfranchi M.D. F.A.C.S. has graciously given me permission to share her well documented research. The two brochures which I found were most helpful are WHAT SMART WOMEN KNOW BEFORE USING THE PILL and THE WHYS OF BREAST CANCER. Both may be read on line. The site also contains nutritional and lifestyle tips. You will also learn why these procedures can unfortunately cause strokes, blood clots and heart attacks. (If this material is helpful to you, I urge you to do what I am doing and share it with important women in your life who are of child bearing age and support these good folks financially.) They do not charge you to look them up on the internet. The bottom line is they have superb well documented research which might save your life and the lives of those whom you love and respect!

THE PILL

Males have laws which prevent them from taking steroids. Shouldn't females have similar protection? The dangerous performance enhancing steroids taken by athletes are male steroid hormonal drugs that build muscle. One of their risks is liver cancer.

Similarly, female steroid hormonal drugs build breast tissue. They not only increase the risk of liver cancer but breast and cervical cancers as well. These powerful steroid drugs are unfortunately taken by millions of teenage girls and women as BIRTH CONTROL PILLS. Should financially motivated drug companies be obligated to report the enclosed dangers of THE PILL with each prescription filled? And to do so in clear language so the average teenager or woman might make an informed choice?

The Center for Disease Control reports that on any given day 85% of the 61 million U.S. women who are of the age to have a child, have used or are using hormonal based birth control pills or methods.

Before taking the pill, smart women will want to weigh the risks and benefits so they can decide what is best for them. The CDC reports that 6-9% of women who faithfully take the pill or use other hormonal enhanced contraceptives such as patches, injections, IUDs or vaginal rings each year will still get pregnant. 17% of women who have abortions were on the pill the month they conceived.

Note: Dr Lanfranchi has 17 footnotes which serious researchers are welcome to investigate for just the brochure on THE PILL. Contrast that with for example groups like Planned Parenthood which make unsupported claims that they provide "safe abortions". (**Should we challenge them to prove it or voluntarily remove this fictitious claim from their websites and advertisements and return donations collected** because they gave an inaccurate description of their service?)
One of the most dangerous practices of groups like Planned Parenthood is that they push the birth control pill with hormonal steroids.

MAJOR SIDE EFFECTS OF TAKING THE PILL

- The pill can make your blood clot. Blood clots in a heart artery can cause a heart attack (myocardial infarction). (20% of those who have their first heart attack die during it.)
- Clots in a brain artery do result in strokes. (CVA)
- Clots in your leg veins, thigh, pelvis or arms can break off and travel through the circulatory system to the lungs and cause a deep venous thrombosis. (DVT) If they lodge in the lungs they cause a fatal pulmonary embolism (PE) 25% of the time. 900,000 Americans die of PE every year. A pulmonary embolism is a blood clot in the lungs. They are known as venous thromboembolisms (VTE). Women

on the pill have a five times greater chance of getting deep venous thrombosis compared to wise women who avoid the pill.

- Women on the pill have two to three times the risk of blood clots.
- New customers who have been on the pill less than a year have three times greater odds of getting a pulmonary embolism compared to wise women who avoid the pill.
- Pulmonary embolism increases by 60 to 80% if the pill had androgenic progestins such as desogestral, gestodene and cyproterone as found in the brands Yal and Yazmin.
- The Ortho-Evra contraception patch has the same percentage of estrogen as the pill, but because it goes through the skin directly into systemic circulation and doesn't go through the liver first it results in 60% higher levels of estrogen.
- No matter how short or long a time a woman on the pill has been using it, she has at least twice the risk of suffering a heart attack. Those who had hypertension had five times the risk. Those who smoked had 12 times the risk. Those who had diabetes had 16 times the risk and those with high cholesterol had 23 times the risk of having a heart attack compared to a non-pill user.
- Meta-analysis occurs when statisticians combine multiple case studies. In this case, the results of 16 studies revealed that the odds of a woman getting a stroke were nearly three times higher if she was on the pill.
- Women on the pill increase the risk of their getting potentially lethal infections such as HIV by 60%. And they were more than twice as likely to transmit HIV to their partners.
- Women on the pill were twice as likely to get infected with HPV (human papilloma virus) which causes cervical cancer.
- The United Nation's International Agency Research of Cancer (IARC) places the pill as a Group 1 Carcinogen for breast, cervical and liver cancers.
- The pill increases the odds of a woman getting cervical cancer by 60% if she uses it for more than five years. Women using it from five to nine years have twice the risk. Woman using the pill for 10 or more years have three times the risk of cervical cancer.

- The pill increases the odds of a woman getting liver cancer by 50%. It also increases the risk of getting benign tumors, hepatic adenomas and nodular hyperplasia (FNH) of the liver. THE LONGER THE PILL IS USED, THE GREATER THE RISKS.
- Long term hormonal contraception was associated with an increase in getting glioma, a type of brain cancer.
- The development of Multiple Sclerosis has been linked to hormonal contraception.
- Women in Denmark who were on the pill had twice the incidence of suicide. (Note: I am Danish.)
- Generally speaking, women on the pill have a higher percentage of incidences of domestic violence.
- In 2000 the National Toxicology Panel labeled estrogen as causing cancer. Metabolites of estrogen directly damage the DNA causing mutations and cancer.
- Since 1975 in-situ breast cancer has increased by 400% in the U.S.
- Some unwise people who like to show off, enjoy playing Russian roulette. They take all but one cartridge out of the cylinder in a revolver, close their eyes, spin it, point it at their head and squeeze the trigger. **Some women who gamble their lives by taking the pill discover that like playing Russian roulette, it is safe until fatal.**

MINOR SIDE EFFECTS OF TAKING THE PILL

They are not life threatening but certainly cause unneeded discomfort and costly inconvenience. They include: weight gain – decreased libido – depression – hypertension – headaches – gall bladder disease – breast tenderness – nausea – mood changes – inter-menstrual spotting – vaginal discharge – visual changes with contact lenses.
MENOPAUSE MEDICATIONS MAY ALSO CONTAIN HARMFUL HORMONES.

Note: There is overlap in the case of women who are approaching menopause. Some of these women unfortunately use meds which also contain hormones to help lessen the discomfort of going through the change of life. Similar dangers lurk and can harm older women as they move on to the next stage of their lives.

CANCERS AND OTHER CHALLENGES

During a woman's lifetime, her breasts are made up of four different types of lobules. Each one is made up of a milk duct and ductiles which form the milk gland where her milk is stored.

- Type 1 lobules exist at birth. 85% of all breast cancers begin here.
- Type 2 lobules are formed during puberty when a young woman's estrogen levels begin to rise. 15% of breast cancers start here.
- Type 3 lobules are formed when a woman's Type 4 lobules stop producing milk and her child is weaned.
- Type 4 lobules initially produce colostrum, a thinner early milk which infants need to get their digestive system up and running and ready for the main course, breast milk.

ONLY TYPE 1 AND TYPE 2 LOBULES ARE VULNERABLE TO CANCER. (On rare occasions a young girl can have a few Type 3 lobules prior to puberty). Some Type 1 lobules will become Type 2 lobules after puberty as the breasts enlarge. At this point the breasts are made up of approximately 75% Type 1 and 25% Type 2 lobules.

By week 20 of a full term (40 week) pregnancy the breasts double in volume, the connective tissue (breast stroma) decreases and the number of lobules increases. DURING THE SECOND HALF OF PREGNANCY, CANCER-VULNERABLE TYPE 1 AND TYPE 2 LOBULES BEGIN TO MATURE INTO CANCER-RESISTANT TYPE 4 LOBULES. Type 4 lobules are capable of producing colostrum and milk that the baby will need. AFTER 32 WEEKS OF PREGNANCY ENOUGH TYPE 4 LOBULES HAVE DEVELOPED SO THAT A MOTHER HAS SIGNIFICANTLY PROTECTED HERSELF AGAINST BREAST CANCER. The benefits are maximized at week 40. By the end of a normal pregnancy 70-90 percent of a mother's breast is composed of cancer-resistant Type 4 lobules.

ONCE THE CHILD IS BORN and the mother has breastfed (or even if she does not breastfeed), TYPE 4 LOBULES REGRESS TO TYPE 3 LOBULES WHICH RETAIN THE EPIGENETIC CHANGES THAT PROTECT AGAINST THE DEVELOPMENT OF CANCER. This epigenetic change involves "down regulation" or "switching off" of lobule reproduction DNA, which thereafter stays permanently switched off and thereby protects against cancer. With each additional pregnancy a woman's risk of breast cancer is lowered an additional 10 percent. THE BOTTOM LINE IS A WOMAN WHO HAS A FULL-TERM PREGNANCY GETS LIFELONG BENEFITS FROM THE EPIGENETIC CHANGES IT PRODUCES IN THE BREAST CELLS AND GAINS EVEN MORE RISK REDUCTION WITH ADDITIONAL BIRTHS AND BREASTFEEDING.

After menopause Type 3 lobules morph into what appear to be Type 1 lobules microscopically. However, the epigenetic changes which have afforded cancer resistance remain. (I urge you to go to www.bcpinstitute.org and click on the Fact Sheet called Breast Development to view illustrations and learn more details. It was my source for this section.) Women should decide if they would be ahead to love and keep their baby and their breasts or to instead end the life of their baby and risk losing their breasts.

STOP READING. Instead please reread the two preceding paragraphs. You will learn the best way to lower the cascading number of breast cancer cases. But this truth needs advocates. Will you be one?

Historical summary: In 1970 only 1 out of 12 women got breast cancer. Roe v. Wade passed in 1973. By 2002 1 out of 7 women had breast cancer. (And some feminists call this legislation a positive and freeing event. Let all pro-choice advocates explain why we should celebrate this cancer statistic!)

Since 1973 invasive breast cancer has risen 40% and non-invasive breast cancer soared 400%!

MEDICAL ASPECTS OF THE PILL

There is another way that the pill kills. A 2017 study of almost half a million Danish women taking the pill showed a 97% increase in suicide attempts and a 208% increase in suicides. The women studied had no prior psychiatric diagnosis or antidepressant use. These women were on various hormonal based contraceptives including the Mirena IUD. The increase occurred two months after starting the pill. (For details go to the Breast Cancer Prevention Institute website www. bcpinstitute.org, click on Brochures and read the one called HOW THE PILL KILLS.) There are 75 million women of reproductive age, 15-45 years old. 82% have taken or are using the pill.

They are also more likely to die a violent death. The longer a woman is on the pill the greater the odds are she will die a violent death. Is this what we want for our young women? The pill kills.

The pill also affects the woman's human partner choice. She is more likely to select someone with similar genetic traits to her own at the DNA loci of the major histocompatibility complex (MHC) genes. Women who marry a man with dissimilar MHC genes have more active and healthier sex lives. If they choose a man with similar genes, they are more likely to have fewer sexual relations, doubt the fidelity of their partner, to be angry and to commit adultery. MHC-similar relationships may have fertility problems and their children are more likely to have genetic defects due to genetic homozygosity/similarity as occurs with close relatives intermarrying.

Furthermore, when two persons have so many similar personality traits it increases the odds of there being intimate partner jealousy, anger and violence. These are the most common causes of nonfatal injury among women and they account for more than a third of women murdered in the United States. Homicide is the most frequent cause of death among pregnant women.

Menstrual periods are lighter because the pill reduces the thickness of the endometrial lining inside the uterus. This complicates things once a woman gets off the pill and desires to have a healthy pregnancy. This makes it more difficult for a fertilized embryo to form a healthy placenta which will implant itself solidly on the healthy wall of the uterus and get the ideal mix of nutrients from the mother. (Tools used in a surgical abortion to scrape the placenta from the uterus and remove a fetus can also cause scarring which can further keep any additional children who are conceived from having optimal nutrition.)

On December 4, 2019, Dr. Michael Lipton, M.D., Ph.D., used a press release through the Radiological Society of North America confirming that current oral contraceptive pill use is associated with women having a significantly smaller essential part of the human brain called the hypothalamus. The hypothalamus regulates mood, menstrual cycles, appetite, sleep cycles, heart rate, temperature, and decreases libido (sex drive). Some women who have taken the pill are surprised to observe, **"I started the pill because I started having sex. Now I'm on the pill and I don't have sex."**

There is an independent risk involved if a woman aborts her first pregnancy. Abortion delays a full term pregnancy for that woman. **FOR EACH YEAR A WOMAN DELAYS HER FIRST PREMENOPAUSAL PREGNANCY, HER RISK OF GETTING BREAST CANCER GOES UP BY 5%.** A woman who has a full term pregnancy at 18 years of age has a 50-75% lower risk of premenopausal breast cancer than a woman who waits until she is 30 to have her first full term pregnancy. The longer a woman waits to have her first child, the greater the odds of having breast cancer.

Can the public always rely on publicly funded agencies such as The National Cancer Institute (NCI) to tell the truth? Although many find it difficult to believe, scientists who get most of their funding from Federal Agencies such as the NCI have admitted to scientific fraud. Physicians are human and are susceptible to the same pressures as other people. Although ideally physicians are trained to be inured to these pressures, sadly not all of us are inure. There is documented evidence of widespread fraud in connection with the National Institute of Health (NIH) funded research (The NCI is part of the NIH).

In 2005 a paper in the British Journal Nature, using anonymous questionnaires, revealed that a statistically significant 15.5% of scientists admitted to "changing the design, methodology or results of a study in response to pressure from a funding source." That funding source was the NIH.

On a related matter women were told the truth about hormone replacement therapy (HRT) and that it increased their risk of getting breast cancer by 26%. In 2002 half of the 37 million women stopped taking HRT. By 2007 there was an 11% reduction in postmenopausal breast cancer attributed to stopping HRT.

The pill uses the same drugs as used in HRT, in more potent formulations. 85% of women of reproductive age have taken or are taking hormonal contraception. Since the early 1970's it is estimated that 30-40% of women have had an abortion by age 40. So it is not surprising that the percentage of women getting cancer has also gone up.

In 2005 the World Health Organization acknowledged that the pill definitely can cause breast cancer. According to a 2011 study by Perkin published in the British Medical Journal, 14.9% of women under age 49 get breast cancer because they took hormonal contraceptives. This is known as an attributable risk. Unfortunately breast cancer patients will likely need help to care for their children, especially during treatment and some will die from it. In 2008 a seven year study of 18,681 women in China revealed that women who experienced one or two abortions increased their odds of getting breast cancer by 151%. Women who had three or more abortions increased the odds of their getting breast cancer by 379%.

Dr. Lanfranchi published her 98 page petition to the FDA on her website www.bcpinstitute.org. Go to the Resources Tab below News and Publications. The petition is also included an unabridged copy of her new book, HEALTH, HORMONES AND CONTRACEPTION. You may freely read, copy or purchase either document on line. She relates how warnings about the pill need to be more readable, be printed in larger and user friendly type rather than being wedged into the product box and published in very small print in language designed for PhD's.

TRIBUTE TO THE BREAST CANCER PREVENTION INSTITUTE (BCPI)

Under the capable leadership of Dr. Lanfranchi, BCPI draws from her 33 years of experience as a surgeon and medical school instructor.

Mission Statement: The Breast Cancer Prevention Institute is a non-profit, 501(c)(3) corporation which educates healthcare professionals and the general public on ways to reduce breast cancer incidence through research, publications, lectures, and the internet.

BCPI was started in 1999 by a scientist and three physicians to educate women and medical professionals. Their website was launched in 2002. Prevention is paramount because even early detection and a high cure rate can't spare a woman the trials of surgery, chemotherapy, radiation and the emotional toll on her loved ones. BCPI is dedicated to educate women and medical professionals on ALL the established, well known and lesser known risks.

Much of the recent surge in breast cancer, especially in young women, is attributable to avoidable risks. Armed with full and accurate information, women can make healthier choices that will reduce their risk of getting breast cancer. These choices also involve lifestyle and dietary strategies.

You will enjoy the website which includes many resources, booklets, brochures, fact sheets, videos, a YouTube video, a semi-annual BCPI report, and news items. I urge you to get on their mailing list and to support them.

Their statistics and facts are very well documented. They rely on readers and supporters to provide for the development of more materials and to maintain their site. Knowledge is power. www.bcpinstitute.org will empower you and reduce your or your loved ones' risk of getting breast cancer. They welcome comments.

Contact Information
Dr. Angela Lanfranchi, MD, FACS
Breast Cancer Prevention Institute
531 US Highway 22 East, Suite 170
Whitehouse Station, NJ 08889 USA
Toll free phone: 1-86-NO CANCER (1-866-622-6237)
Telephone: 908-745-8451
Email: info@bcpinstitute.org

ABORTION, NURSING AND BREAST CANCER

An amazing statistic follows.

Why is it that since abortion was legalized in the United States in 1973 the rate of breast cancer has soared? There were an estimated 68,000 new cases of breast cancer among U.S. women in 1970 (Silverberg and Grant 1970). By 2014, there was a 242 percent increase (232,670) in new cases of female breast cancer (Siegel, Zou, and Jemal 2014). From1970 to 2014 the U.S. population increased 56.8 percent (203,392,031 to 318,892,100). **Thus, the rate of increase in female breast cancer has been more than 4-fold** (i.e., 4.26-fold) the increase in the U.S. population during the same period. (Source: The Linacre Quarterly, August 2014: https://www.ncbi.nlm.nih.gov/pmc/articles/PMC4135458/). In 1981 researchers in southern California found that if the first pregnancy was aborted, breast cancer increased by 140%. In 1989 the New York State Department of Health documented that **any induced abortion increase breast cancer risk by 90%. If a woman had two abortions the risk increased by 300%.** In 1994 a study in Seattle showed **abortions done on minors increased breast cancer risk by 150%.** This is one reason states should require parents be notified if their underage daughter is getting an abortion. They could warn their daughter that she would be more susceptible to getting breast cancer. Many Jews and liberal Protestants permit abortion. **Jewish women have a 2.8 times higher rate of breast cancer than Catholics according to a multinational study in 1983.** Liberal Protestants have a higher risk of breast cancer in Canada compared to Catholic women. Should women who elect to have an abortion be required to read these statistics? (We thank Lutherans for Life for supplying many of these statistics.)

THE STATISTIC ABORTIONISTS MUST ABSOLUTELY REFUTE - OR STOP CLAIMING ABORTION IS SAFE

Enter into your search engine "Howard University Study 1993 Black American women getting breast cancer". We read, "A highly significant 1993 Howard University Study showed that Black American women over age 50 are 4.7 times more likely to get breast cancer if they had any abortions compared to Black American women who had not had abortions." {www.blackgenocide.org. Life Education And Resource Network (LEARN) -- Northeast Chapter.} Let any abortionist who claims that there are no increases in breast cancer when one has an abortion please be so kind as to refute this specific statistic. Or else apologize for their inaccurate statement! **This is a specific challenge. I invite the abortion community to send their replies to me in care of my publisher or stop claiming that abortion is safe.**

Now let's review a key factor. It can take 10 or more years before the tiny initial cancer cell has grown large enough for it to be identified by feeling the cancer lump or seeing evidence of it on a mammogram. So a large percentage of women who are checked to see whether or not they have breast cancer can have it, but it is too small to be discovered. The most important age category of women who are diagnosed with having breast cancer are those who have had abortions more than ten years before they are tested!!! Some deceptive or poorly trained pro-choice advocates conveniently report that because there is no verifiable sign of cancer during the ten years after the women had their abortion, therefore the abortion did not harm them. This is an unacceptable and very possibly lethal misdiagnosis.

If you are being pitched by the sales person at an abortion facility that abortion is safe, please show them this entry and have them defend their claim that they offer safe abortions. Note: The sooner a woman with breast cancer is diagnosed, the greater the chance that it can be successfully treated!

ALL BLACK LIVES MATTER (FROM CONCEPTION TO NATURAL DEATH)

Perhaps Black Lives Matter should start a subsidiary organization with this title. Many think it's strange that when a single black man, George Floyd was murdered, there were riots and destruction and looting of property. **But when abortionists kill 1,452 black babies a day in America, groups like Black Lives Matter never burn down an abortion clinic or launch complaints at this injustice.** I have no doubt that black leaders will come up with a plan to correct this inequitable situation.

According to protectingblacklife.org, "A 2010 census reveals that Planned Parenthood is targeting minority neighborhoods. **79% of their surgical abortion facilities are located within walking distance of Black American or Hispanic/ Latino neighborhoods.**" Let's summarize the racist Roots of Planned Parenthood with the words of its founder Margaret Sanger ("Pivot of Civilization"). **Concerning blacks, immigrants and indigents, she says they are, "…human weeds, reckless breeders, spawning…human beings who should have never been born." Which secular or Christian black groups are protesting this quote and the placement of abortion facilities in minority neighborhoods?**

38TH & CHICAGO – WHAT WENT WRONG

I have been trying to focus on what went wrong when four police officers failed to safely arrest, restrain and bring the suspect who lost his life into custody. (Peace be to his memory and may his family and friends know we see their tears, genuinely care and share their sorrow.)

IT WAS A TRAINING PROBLEM. IF THEY WOULD HAVE BEEN PROPERLY TRAINED THIS WOULD NEVER HAVE HAPPENED. I suggest we consider that, **"Maybe the senior officer whom God wanted to train the four policemen was aborted."**

For sure when someone is in a restraint and multiple officers are present, one of them should have the specific assignment of monitoring and taking notes on the prisoner's breathing (how many breaths per minute. Was the breathing abnormal?) It was totally unacceptable that no one observed that his breathing stopped. There needs to be a protocol about what to do when a prisoner's breathing is abnormal or stops. Another officer should be responsible for and possibly responding to what the prisoner says. Were the officers conforming to having their body cameras on?

Law enforcement, military personnel and elected officials working at every level to protect and serve our citizens should be properly trained. May every person, be they following the laws or considering breaking them to send a message to our leaders, be able to express themselves in safety without harming people or damaging property. May all lives be they preborn or born, MAY ALL LIVES MATTER. And may we consider the personnel shortages which will occur each time an innocent child in the womb has his or her life ended. Let every child be wanted, nurtured, valued, respected, and most of all loved.

Perhaps you are thinking, Dale, this doesn't concern you. Let me tell you I take what happened on 38th and Chicago in South Minneapolis personally. Why? I was confirmed in Calvary Lutheran Church, one block south of the site of the tragic unnecessary murder. My folks and all four of my grandparents also worshipped there. What happened occurred on my turf. So I have skin in the game. Don't disrespect my efforts to analyze what went wrong! Give my theory full consideration.

ACHILLES HEAL – DEMOCRATIC PARTY

I have a friend, who when he turned 18 decided to attend the Democratic caucus. He was excited to participate in the political process and went to the Democratic precinct caucus in Shakopee, MN. The chairman said, "The floor is open to propose items for consideration in our platform. Anyone is welcome to present them."

He stood up and said, "I wish to propose a pro-life plank." Those present shouted him down and told him there is no way they would ever accept any pro-life platform ideas. They wouldn't even let him read the proposal so they could vote on it.

I just learned about this. Immediately I asked him, "So what did you do?" He said, "I left the Democratic pro-choice party. I have been a proud conservative pro-life Republican ever since."

"As you do not know how the Spirit comes to the bones in the womb of a woman with child, so you do not know the work of God who makes everything" (Ecclesiastes 11:5). *"I am wiser than all my teachers, because I think about your rules. I have more understanding than the elders, because I follow your orders. I have avoided every evil way so I could obey your word"* (Psalm 119:99-101).

BREAST FEEDING AND BREAST CANCER

A 2009 study published in The Archives of Internal Medicine reported that among 60,000 women with a family history of breast cancer, women who breast fed reduced the chances of their getting breast cancer before the onset of menopause by nearly 60%. (Research dangerous chemicals in cow's milk.)

A study of 150,000 women published in The Lancet in 2002 found that for every one year of breast feeding for an entire year, whether it was for one or multiple children, the risk of getting breast cancer was reduced by 4.3% compared to women who never breast fed.

One theory as to why this happens is that women who breast feed have fewer menstrual cycles throughout their lives. And therefore less exposure to estrogen which has been shown to fuel some types of breast cancer. 78% of all breast cancers are fueled by estrogen. Another theory is that the breast cells of women who breastfeed are protected from mutations which contribute to getting the disease. https://www.glamcheck. com/health/2012/06/r-breast-cancer-how-are-they-related. **It also reduces the risk of a baby girl who was nursed from eventually getting breast cancer. In addition, children who are nursed have fewer allergies.**

BENEFITS TO THE INFANT

I would like to commend WebMD for much of the following information. What are the benefits of breast feeding your baby? Breast milk provides ideal nutrition for newborns. **It has a nearly perfect blend of vitamins, protein and fat - everything your baby needs to grow.** It is more easily digested than infant formula. The antibodies contained in breast milk strengthen your baby to successfully fight off **viruses (think coronavirus)** and **bacteria**. It reduces the risk of having **asthma** or **allergies**. An infant breastfed for the first six months will have fewer **ear infections, respiratory illnesses**, bouts of **diarrhea, trips to the doctor** or **hospitalizations**. It is linked to **higher IQ scores** in later childhood. Additionally, the **closeness, skin to skin touching** and **eye contact** strengthen the bond between mom and child and increase their feeling of **security**. Breastfed infants are more likely to gain the right amount of **weight** rather than becoming overweight. A baby who falls asleep drinking from a bottle of cow's milk is more likely to have **cavities in their teeth**. Breast feeding helps prevent **SIDS (Sudden Infant Death Syndrome)**. It reduces the odds of someone eventually getting **diabetes or becoming obese**. In addition, if a mother nurses her child, it lowers the odds of her child having medical problems such as allergies and of a girl child getting breast cancer in the future and the mother getting breast cancer. Infants are not capable of safely digesting whole milk from the store during the infants' first six months. Infant formula is better. Breast milk is best. For the first year of his life, my son and daughter-in-law wisely obtained donated breast milk for their adopted son.

BENEFITS FOR MOM

Breast feeding **burns calories** and helps a mom **lose her pregnancy weight faster**. It **releases oxytocin**, a hormone which **helps the uterus return to its pre-pregnancy size**. It **reduces uterine bleeding** after birth. It lowers the risk of **breast and ovarian cancer** and possibly **of osteoporosis**. Mom doesn't have to take the **time** and **expense** to warm and prepare a bottle and can instead use the **time to bond** with her baby. THEREFORE INSTEAD OF HAVING AN ABORTION WHICH WILL INCREASE THE ODDS OF HER GETTING BREAST CANCER, BY BIRTHING AND NURSING HER LOVELY BABY, SHE WILL LOWER HER RISK OF GETTING BREAST CANCER!

HOW NOT BREAST FEEDING PROVED TO BE AN UNWISE CHOICE FOR MY MOTHER

When my sister who is two years younger than me was born, mom had serious bleeding problems. Her doctor was unable to stop her from bleeding. She was even placed on her back and a board was placed over her uterus and fastened on both sides to the bed. To save her from bleeding to death, she unfortunately had to have a complete hysterectomy while in her 20's. (We do not know for sure if nursing would have helped her to stop the bleeding, but had her doctor known that in general it does reduce the odds of bleeding, I am confident he would have prescribed she do so.) This unfortunate incident ended my parents' dream of having a large family. But their love for young people continued. My parents reached out to them in interesting ways. For example, Juliet Nurse from South America was a gifted black art student at the Minneapolis Institute of Art. Unfortunately she had severe scoliosis. Her spine was so severely bent, her organs were in danger of shutting down. Her classmates had a big art sale to pay for the surgery. A physician donated his services. But she needed to be in a body cast for a year. My folks let her live with them during that time. Mom was second in her nursing class at Minneapolis Fairview Hospital. She explained the reason she wasn't at the top of her nursing class was because the girl who was first never dated. Mom had an active social life and was actually engaged twice prior to Dad's capturing her heart. To wash Juliet's hair, they laid her on the kitchen counter and used the sink sprayer. Juliet's mom had died. When her father visited her from South America, and she met people, she would say, "This is my father" and pointing to mom, "And this is my mother." So I have a black sister. Isn't that great? She would go on to marry and have a lovely daughter who became Miss British Guiana. They visited our family every few years. When mom was a student nurse, one of her large muscular patients would sometimes have a violent incident. It would take three men to hold him down. When mom was caring for him, she had a prayer in her heart and never once did he become violent. When the Lord lives in our hearts, He empowers us. Who wouldn't want this blessing?

On a personal note, neither my sister nor I were breast fed. From birth my sister Dodie had severe eczema. It was only when her pediatrician suggested that my mom buy her goat's milk that Dodie's eczema disappeared. When we were in grade school an allergist tested us. Scratch tests include being injected with samples of various foods and plants. Then the size of the swelling is charted on a one to ten. My mom and I were in the waiting room while my sister was being administered tests for food allergies. The allergist rushed into the waiting room and instructed my mother to come with him. When he had injected my sister with "beets", she had a cardiac arrest! With mom watching, he injected a stimulant into my sister's heart. Thankfully it successfully restarted!

My sister who was in second grade laughed it off with the comment, "Not to worry. I never liked beets anyway." My biggest allergy was to the plant goldenrod. When I finished kindergarten, my father took a teaching job and our family moved from California to Minnesota. Hay fever caused my eyes to tear. Some mornings the tears had hardened in my eyelashes so I couldn't open my eyes. Mom would apply a hot wash cloth to them, dissolving enough of the deposits so I could open my eyes and rinse them and my eyelashes with warm water. My allergies to the pollen in the autumn air were so severe, on the advice of my allergist, my folks had me move to Duluth, Minnesota, where the air coming off Lake Superior is pollen free. I stayed in a Lutheran Children's Home there until the first frost. Then I returned to live with my family in Minneapolis. As I grew older and later had prayers for healing, my allergies gradually diminished.

The theory is that when a mother nurses her infant, the infant benefits from the development of her immune system. When a woman is lactating, carcinogens which exist in the air are unable to store themselves in the fat tissue of the breasts. So nursing helps protect the mother from environmental dangers such as air pollution. *Let Global Warming advocates therefore campaign against abortion and for breast feeding!*

On a personal note, **when I was an adolescent, I speculated what might be the most beautiful sight I would ever see during my lifetime.** I imagined it would be my future wife nursing our child. When this happened, I realized I had imagined correctly. Did you know the distance at which a newborn infant's eyes focus match the space between a nursing child and her mom's eyes? What a tremendous bonding opportunity! Finally, nursing put my wife in a romantic mood. So I encouraged my wife to nurse my son.

(Legislative recommendation: a form indicating the dangers to a mother having an abortion needs to be written. Then before an abortion facility can end the life of a child, the mother should always be required to sign this form indicating she recognizes these medical

and emotional risks. Signing the form would not mean the mother surrendered her right to litigate against the abortionist if the procedure injured her. The facility would forever be held to stand behind their claim that abortion was safe and legal. **I would like there to be no statute of limitations on malpractice related to abortion procedures.)**

You might enjoy reading a couple of additional scriptures regarding breasts: *"Even by the God of thy father, Who shall help thee; and by the Almighty, Who shall bless thee with blessings of heaven above, blessings of the deep that lieth under, blessings of the breasts, and of the womb"* (Genesis 49:25), *"But Thou art He that took me out of the womb: **Thou didst make me hope when I was upon my mother's breasts"*** (Psalms 22:9). *"Can a mother forget the baby at her breast and have no compassion on the child she has borne? Though she may forget, I will not forget you"* (Isaiah 49:15), *"Gather the people, sanctify the congregation, assemble the elders, gather the children, and those that suck the breasts: let the bridegroom go forth of his chamber, and the bride out of her closet"* (Joel 2:16).

PEOPLE FOR THE ETHICAL TREATMENT OF ANIMALS (PETA)

PETA protects animals from being treated cruelly. During 2019 they published solicitations for rewards of five thousand dollars. The first was for helping to locate and arrest a person who cruelly tied one or more firecrackers to the leg of a cat. No doubt when they went off the injuries to the cat were painful and substantial.

The second reward for five thousand dollars was set up to locate and arrest a person who burned a dog. A third five thousand dollar reward was for someone who threw poisoned meat into the yard of a two year old Shiatsu who had seizures and died. "This little dog undoubtedly endured agonizing pain and terror as her body began to seize and shut down," says PETA Vice President Colleen O'Brien. Those with information about this case should call Crime Stoppers of Nevada at

702-385-5555." **May I suggest PETA extend their goal of protecting innocent pets to include innocent unborn children?** Isn't it ironic that many of the same public who applaud the excellent work PETA does protecting animals usually remain uninterested in protecting innocent unborn children?

Susan B. Anthony, a pioneer in the women's movement, was passionately pro-life. Anthony held both men and women responsible for abortion because it hurts women and "murders" a child. She wrote, "…No matter what the motive, love of ease or desire to save the innocent unborn from suffering, the woman is awfully guilty who commits the deed (abortion). It will burden her conscience in life. It will burden her soul in death: But oh! **Thrice guilty is he who, for selfish gratification, heedless of her prayers, indifferent to her fate, drove her to the desperation which impels her to the crime."**

SIGNIFICANT STATISTICS AND RACIAL DISCRIMINATION

These abortion statistics primarily come from the internet search July 2019:
- Worldwide since 1980: 1,544,529,959
- Worldwide during 2018: 24,823,148
- United States abortions since 1973 and Roe vs. Wade: 61,514,499
- By Planned Parenthood since 1970: 8,499,451
- In 2018 abortions due to rape or incest: 5,553
- "Several years ago, when 17,000 aborted babies were found in a dumpster outside a pathology laboratory in Los Angeles, CA, approximately 13,500 were observed to be black." (Erma Clardy Craven, deceased social worker and civil rights leader)
- In the United States during 2018 25.9% of abortions were performed after the sixteenth week of gestation. Currently after 16 weeks gestation America has 27,478 annual abortions.

The Pharmacists For Life organization estimates that **THERE HAVE BEEN APPROXIMATELY 250 MILLION AMERICAN**

BABIES ABORTED CHEMICALLY SINCE 1973!!! (http://www.pfli.org/)
In 1984 abortions after 20 weeks were 30,000 according to the center for disease control. 4,000 of these were in the third trimester.
The suction device used to destroy an infant growing in the womb is much more powerful than a home vacuum cleaner. Colorado **abortionist Warren Hern, who does late term abortions reports,** "...the emotional turmoil that the procedure inevitably wreaks on physicians and staff... There is no possibility of denial of an act of destruction by the operator...**The sensations of dismemberment flow through the forceps like an electric current**...Some part of our cultural and perhaps even biological heritage recoils at a destructive operation on a form similar to our own..." **(Meeting of American Association of Planned Parenthood Physicians OB-GYN News,** 1978 Dr. & Mrs. J.C. Willke in their book, ABORTION QUESTIONS AND ANSWERS p.19). ASK YOUR ABORTIONIST, "WHAT IS DR. HERN SAYING? HAVE YOU EVER HAD SECOND THOUGHTS ABOUT YOUR PROFESSION?"
According to the Guttmacher Institute in 2017 there were 890,000 abortions in the United States. In 1996 there were 1,360,000 abortions. Washington D.C. aborts 37% of their children. New Jersey aborts 32%. North Dakota aborts 4%. Wyoming aborts 2%.

WHICH BLACK GROUPS DEMAND THE CLOSING OF ALL ABORTION FACILITIES BECAUSE THE FOUNDER OF PLANNED PARENTHOOD WAS SO PREJUDICED? What else did the founder of Planned Parenthood have to say? Margaret Sanger, founder of Planned Parenthood wanted *"more children from the fit, less from the unfit."* (BIRTH CONTROL REVIEW, VOL. 3, NO.5, May 1919, p.2) In January 2020 Priests For Life reported that **78% of Planned Parenthood abortion clinics are in or next to minority communities.** Planned Parenthood's founder Margaret Sanger designed The Negro Project to sterilize (unknown to them) black women and others she deemed undesirable to society. She explained, *"Colored people are like human weeds and need to be exterminated."* **Pro-choice**

founders and leaders admit they want to limit the number of black children being born. If you doubt present Planned Parenthood leaders want to reduce the number of black children being born, PROPOSE THAT ALL CLINICS IN PREDOMINANTLY BLACK NEIGHBORHOODS BE MOVED INTO PREDOMINANTLY WHITE NEIGHBORHOODS. Please contact me with the results. (Some black organizations make the case that because of slavery, black people should receive reparations. **Why don't these folks expand their request for financial justice through reparations to include Planned Parenthood's deliberate goal of reducing the number of black children being born?** See also usabortionclock.org.)

On November 28, 2018 cnsnews.com reported, **"Although black Americans comprise only 13.4% of the United States population they accounted for 36.6% of abortions."** This statistic is almost identical to the percentage of abortions (36.9%) that year among white Americans who make up 76.6% of our population.

With 1/3 of all abortions in America being performed on black women the abortion industry has received over $4 billion from the black community.

Since 1973 18,454,350 black babies were aborted. On average 1,452 black babies are aborted every day in America.

In Georgia where our black friends make up 32.2% of the population and whites make up 60.8%, black women had 62.4% of abortions and white women only had 24.7%. In New York City, more black children were aborted than were born alive.

IMPORTANT STATISTICS PRIMARILY FROM LUTHERANS FOR LIFE

FACT: California, New Hampshire and Maryland do not report abortion statistics.

FACT: In 2018 abortion killed 876,000 unborn children.

FACT: (in some states) Abortion is legal throughout the entire nine months of pregnancy. 8 to 10 percent of abortions in America occur in the last two trimesters.

FACT: At 12 weeks of age, the unborn child has all the body parts (nerves, spinal cord, thalamus) needed to experience pain. Brain waves have been present for 6 weeks and a heartbeat for 8 weeks.

FACT: Repeat abortions: The Guttmacher Institute, Volume 10, Issue 2 by Susan A. Cohen reports that, "About half of all U. S. women having an abortion have had one previously". (After their abortions, 25% of the women are unable to conceive again. Should abortionists offer to sterilize women and/or men who come for repeat abortions?)

FACT: A recent obstetrical study listed abortion as the 6th most common cause of maternal deaths. The Center for Disease Control, which conducted the study, admitted that maternal deaths due to abortion may be under-reported by as much as 50%.

FACT: Another study tells that 81% of aborted women report *preoccupation* with the aborted child; 73% report flashbacks; 69% report "craziness" after abortion; 54% report nightmares; 35% report visitations from the aborted child; 23% report hallucinations related to abortion.

FACT: Since the Revolutionary War, **1.2 million Americans have died in armed conflict. (In World War I, 116,708 American military personnel died from all causes. In World War II over 405,000 Americans gave their lives in the conflict. In Desert Storm 293 Americans died.)** Since 1973, when abortion-on-demand was legalized by the Supreme Court **over 61 million babies have died by abortion. Add to this statistic the 250 million who are chemically aborted** (as reported by Pharmacists For Life).

FACT: There are 426 abortions for every 1,000 live births in the U.S.

LEGISLATIVE SUGGESTIONS

The medical people who end innocent lives are stealing money from their peers. These unborn victims and their children and their children's children would have paid for health care for years and years...and multiple generations. (If the aborted children would have lived, they would have incurred medical expenses and also bought things from merchants. Should the medical people and merchants sue abortionists for depriving them of income?) Abortionists have caused grade schools to close, teachers and staff to be laid off. Should educators sue abortionists? How much are the abortionists taking from their pockets? **Abortion wraps a heavy chain of financial devastation around our swimming nation.**

The federal debt per citizen on March, 2021 was $84,920. The gross federal debt was $28 trillion. (Source: https://www. usdebtclock.org/)

RATIO OF WORKERS TO RETIRED PEOPLE

Roe vs. Wade was passed in 1973. The ratio of workers supporting retired people in 1945 was 41.9 to each retiree, 1950-16.5, 1960-5.1, 1970-3.7, 2010-2.9, 2013-2.8. (Source: https://www.ssa.gov/history/ratios.html) Projecting into the future, according to the Social Security Administration compiled by the Peter G. Peterson Foundation, by 2030 the ratio will drop to 2.4.

The single biggest problem is that the ratio of workers to the number of people who want to retire is permanently damaged. Other factors affecting this ratio include families waiting longer to have their first child and that people are living longer and fewer people are getting married. Retirements are postponed. Some project that a new specialty of attorneys will be setting up shop, starting with medical malpractice suits for physical and emotional damage done by the mercenary medical pro-choice crowd. For starters, each and every physician and abortion facility that has been sued for malpractice by their patients and lost....should be required to post a *malpractice scorecard* on their website so all can see their weaknesses.... what they did which caused them to lose money and the amount of each settlement. Individuals who were promised things by their abortionists....and lied to....need to have their day in court. Should abortion providers be required to justify their claim that they are providing "safe abortions"? Why shouldn't they **go point by point and speak to the dangers of abortion as described in this book? If they fail to do so, we respectfully ask them to apologize and withdraw the bogus claim that they provide "safe abortions" and cease performing them. Should someone who tampers with a death certificate be allowed to keep their medical license? Perhaps we should research all death certificates of women who have had an abortion and died within the next twelve months to see if their cause of death is blackened out. If it is blacked out or suspicious, investigate.**

MY POLITICAL TAKE ON THE PRESENT SITUATION

Although I was pre-med during part of my college experience and my wife had degrees in nursing and anesthesia, I am only a lay person with no formal medical training. If you were to get the opinion of just one person regarding whether abortion was right or wrong....what credentials would such a person have? I nominate the name of Bernard Nathanson, MD. In his autobiography, THE HAND OF GOD, he describes his background p.5, **"I am one of those who helped usher in this barbaric age. I worked hard to make abortion legal, affordable, and available on demand. In 1968, I was one of the three founders of the National Abortion Rights Action league. I ran the largest abortion clinic in the United States, and as its director I oversaw tens of thousands of abortions.** I have performed thousands myself. How could this have happened? How could I have done this?" Dr. Nathanson explains his father's background, **"My father, whom I loved deeply and loathed equally deeply... was a formidable, dominant force in my life and in many** lives...forged the ruthless, nihilistic, pagan attitudes and beliefs that finally drove me to unleash with a handful of co-conspirators--the abortion monster." Dr. Nathanson's father's father was a pharmacist who contracted tuberculosis. It was the AIDS of that day. In order to give his body a chance to heal, he was sent to a sanitarium in Colorado, with the hope that the clear fresh air would rejuvenate his body. While there, he learned that, "his wife and children were in a state of near starvation owing to the allocation of most of their available funds to finance his stay in Colorado. Very shortly thereafter, he hanged himself in his closet, the better to divert the funds into food for his children."

FALSE STATISTICS USED IN PASSING ROE VS. WADE - WHY WEREN'T THESE STATISTICS CHALLENGED IN 1973?

Dr. Bernard Nathanson, in his bestseller ABORTING AMERICA admits that **the reported five to ten thousand women per year dying from back-alley abortions was "totally false."** In his book he explained that he and others circulated these false figures in 1972 in order to bring about legal abortion.

In 1972 only 39 abortion-related deaths were officially reported. Admittedly, if back-alley abortions are not reported, deaths connected with them certainly wouldn't be. Wouldn't the misstatement of these statistics mandate Roe vs. Wade be re-litigated? (See also p.81 of the book POST ABORTION TRAUMA by Jeanette Vought.)

We who love life applaud that Roe has been overturned. Note also that *Norma Leah Nelson, the person who was used as the plaintiff in Roe vs. Wade regrets being used in this way and wishes the decision had never been made. That plaintiff is now vocally pro-life!*

A PRO-LIFE INDIVIDUAL'S AGGREGIOUS MISTAKE

We who are pro-life are also against taking the life of any abortionist. It should be noted that on October 26, 1998 abortionist doctor Barnett Stepian was senselessly killed. We condemn this act!! We pray for his grieving family and offer them our sympathy.

WHERE DO YOU WANT TO SPEND ETERNITY?

If you, dear reader, are involved in the abortion industry, we invite you to join the growing ranks of former abortionists who have resigned their positions with cause, and become pro-life. Hebrews 9:27 clearly states, *"It is given to man once to die and then comes judgment."*

*"Yea, to Him shall all the proud of the earth bow down; **before Him shall bow all who go down to the dust, and he who cannot keep himself alive.** Posterity shall serve Him; men shall tell of the Lord to the coming generation, and proclaim His deliverance to a people yet unborn, that He has performed it"* (Psalm 22: 29-31). *God will judge you for your career choice. We don't wish you to spend eternity regretting your wrong choices.* Keep reading this document and you can discover a way out of your bad choices and unwise lifestyle. We offer a hand up. There is an old story that Satan asked his demons, "How can we get people to not worry about having to pay for their sinful choices?" The first said, "We can tell them there is no hell." The second said, "We can tell them they deserve the financial and pleasurable benefits of their sinful choices." The third had his suggestion accepted when he said, "We can tell them that there is no rush to act on these facts." *We see every pro-choice advocate as a potential champion for life.* What if Ronald Reagan, George Bush and Doctor Bernard Nathanson had lost their lives because of their one time views? What if the Christians in Jerusalem would have killed Saul following his being in charge of the stoning of Stephen, the church's first martyr? (Acts 7:84) Saul was renamed the

apostle Paul, author of much of the New Testament. When you finish using your computer to watch Jesusfilm.org which uses as its script Luke's gospel, read the book of Acts also written by the physician, Dr. Luke. You will learn how the Messiah transformed the murderer Saul into the Apostle Paul. It documents what happened to the believers after the resurrected Messiah returned to heaven. **We pro-life folks basically see you, our pro-choice friends as our future allies, and wish you all the best.** We care not only about the well being of your patients, we care about you. (If you doubt this, and pro-life counselors arrive at your facility hoping to talk with your clients, offer to meet with them privately for coffee or a meal. Take the initiative and befriend them.) Boldly introduce yourself to the resources in this book.

CONVOLUTED LOGIC – POWER STRUGGLE

One reason <u>feminists were angry</u> with strong men was because the <u>men unfairly used their strength to force their will on the women</u>.

But today, <u>some women who are pro-choice are doing the same thing to innocent unborn children. They are using their superior strength</u> to kill innocent unborn children. And many do so shamelessly, with pride.

Two men were down in a ditch, digging it and making $10.00 per hour. They were being supervised by a man who did no work, but only told them what to do. He was standing next to the ditch leaning against a steel column and making $20.00 per hour.

One of the men climbed up and asked his supervisor, "Why are you making twice what we earn?" His supervisor explained, "Because I am smarter than you." The ditch digger said, "Prove it." His supervisor placed his hand on the steel column and said, "Hit my hand." The ditch digger swung hard to do so. But right before he made contact, the supervisor pulled his hand away. And the ditch digger smashed his fist painfully into the steel pier.

When the ditch digger reentered the ditch, his partner asked, "So what happened?" The ditch digger put his good hand on the front of his face and told his partner. "Hit my hand."

One main reason some women say abortion is OK is that they believe "a woman has the right to control her own body". They identify their baby as part of their own body. Let's carry this argument forward. Everyone would agree that it's wrong to kill a mother. So if an abortionist kills an unborn child should that abortionist be prosecuted for killing a mother? Perhaps it is time to let the courts decide if an abortionist is guilty of ending the life of the mother?

When you think about it, **abortionists are stronger and smarter than women in a crisis pregnancy.** Is it fair that they use their superior power to talk women into sacrificing the lives of their unborn children and risking their health when they invite abortionists to give them abortions? And to think that some women even ask the abortionists to do so an additional time? 45% of all women who have an abortion have had one before. (Source: Journal of Women's Health, January 1, 2018, https://www.ncbi.nlm.nih.gov/pmc/articles/PMC5771530/)

180 DEGREES

What I'd really like to see is for abortion clinics to make two changes. **FIRST, stop doing abortions and instead help women in crisis or normal pregnancy situations to deliver full term radiantly healthy children.** The upgraded counseling center would provide complete pro-life OB/GYN services for women. They would gradually add complete pediatric care for children. They would provide services for parents with post abortion syndrome (PAS) including resource and support groups, they could view https://www. silentnomoreawareness.org/, 412-749-0455. They are interested in increasing their bottom line. I project **over time my plan would increase abortion clinics' annual income substantially. (**They could rehire employees who resigned because they didn't want to do abortions anymore.) Based on the most recent data from usda.gov, the Consumer Expenditures Survey, in 2015, a family will spend approximately $12,980 annually per child in a middle-income ($59,200-$107,400), two-child, married-couple family. If they're smart, abortion clinics could capture a nice percentage of that $12,980 annual sum. It makes more business sense to do this rather than to be satisfied with a fee for an abortion. Now their clients usually just pay a onetime fee with the exception of the ones who come back for additional abortions. Plus some of those profits are lost because of malpractice suits. I also propose that they let all of their salaried employees vote on accepting my proposal by taking a confidential vote. **Each pro-choice facility would poll their staff and abide by the results.** Not all facilities would agree at first, but a repeat vote could be taken quarterly. When income from the sites which switched their policies soared, other sites would follow. This way God could bless their staff and supporters. Forgiveness for breaking God's Ten Commandments could be given. And **employees would receive the benefits of life with the Lord now and eternity with Him and loved ones in heaven in the future.**

$600 - $2,500

My personal view is that if a doctor or crisis pregnancy counselor, be they pro-choice or pro-life helps a woman in a crisis pregnancy to give their child up for adoption, that person or organization should be paid $600 when the adoption is completed. (I wish to compliment an interview I heard with one abortion provider. He admitted that he was not in it primarily to benefit a woman in a crisis pregnancy. He admitted that he was in it for the money. The person interviewing asked, "If instead of getting $600 for doing an abortion, if you were given $1,200 to talk the woman into birthing her baby and giving it up for adoption, what would you do?" The abortionist said, "I would take the $1,200.")

We are who pro-life should use this knowledge to set things up so abortionists would make more money guiding women to give their baby up for adoption than they would net if they sold a woman an abortion.

I also believe that a woman who gives her child up for adoption should be paid $2,500 tax free when the adoption is finalized. If the mother committed to give up the child to a specific couple or person it might be alright for the mother to ask for additional financial assistance during the balance of her pregnancy.

Every time a child is saved from abortion, we can anticipate the ratio of workers to people who are retired will be improved. And the beauty of it is it will cost the taxpayers nothing. The same clinic which encouraged the woman to birth instead of to abort her baby would be the obvious place a woman would come to birth her child and obtain pediatric care. I would like to see legislators from all parties co-sponsor such a bill and welcome these children into our homes and country with love and open arms. K-12 schools could be reopened, teachers and support staff could be rehired. Financial surpluses are certainly preferable to promising retirement funds with no hope of ever being able to supply them. It is irresponsible to keep printing money and mortgaging the future of our young people. A side benefit would be the avoidance of malpractice lawsuits initiated by women who are harmed by abortionists.

How about legislating that pro-life facilities get a fair share of government funding to help their clients? Perhaps an equal amount of funding for each client that abortion businesses get for each of their abortion clients? Let us keep in mind pro-life folks increase the amount of income the government needs to fund social security and provide workers for businesses. So the government will reap a rich reward for funds directed to pro-life advocacy. **What reward do our tax dollars designated for abortion clinics bring us?!** Project these statistics out 10, 20, 50 years, etc. then decide if my recommendations are morally and fiscally sound.

SECOND, I would also like to see all abortion clinics stop all involvement with Comprehensive Sex Ed (CSE). See cplaction.com for details. A summary of their unwise programs is located in the Resource Section of this book. The Child Protection League is an exceptional resource leading the fight to combat CSE. 888-538-3188. Get on their mailing list. Vote out all elected officials who support their toxic programs. If any government funds have been given CSE, cancel their support. Figure out ways to present logical arguments to all students who have been programmed to accept their dangerous viewpoints so students can be reoriented to traditional Godly values supported by America's founding fathers. (Some former abortion providers admit that one reason abortion clinics are promoting CSE is that they want more teenagers to become pregnant. They hope these teenagers would come in to buy an abortion.)

SHORTAGE OF INFANTS, SURPLUS OF PARENTS WANTING TO ADOPT – CREATIVE ALTERNATIVE TO ADOPTING A NEWBORN

There simply are not enough babies for those who desire them. I personally know of one couple who desired to adopt an infant. When they discovered there was a 10 year waiting list for one, they discontinued their quest.

To couples who desire to adopt, I suggest you research becoming foster parents. There are churches that partnered with foster care programs and successfully encouraged their members to adopt a large percentage of the kids in foster care in their communities. Foster parents are **screened** and **trained**. They are **paid** to invite children to live with them for a limited period. Appropriate **supervision** and **support** are given to foster parents so they can be successful meeting the needs of those in their care. (My son and his wife genuinely enjoyed foster parenting 13 different kids.) If foster parents find a child who seems like a good fit, they can apply to adopt that child. **Older children also need loving parents**. I am a landlord. One of my most rewarding experiences as a landlord concerned one of my tenants who was a Native American foster parent. She cared for children of Indian families while their parents were in treatment. Gradually, the parents' visitation rights were increased. And most won their children back.

The costs of adopting a foster child are minimal. The biggest expense for a foster care adoption is the home study, which can cost anywhere from $1,000 to $5,000. If the adoption is completed through an agency there may be required agency fees that an adoptive family must also pay. (https://consideringadoption.com › adopting › foster-care-adoption-costs)

I have terrific news for you prospective parents who hope to adopt a child. In round figures there are 430,000 children in the United States who are in foster care. Approximately 125,000 of them are eligible to be adopted today. So how can you learn about foster children in your state? First, what my son and his wife did was search the internet for Minnesota Adoption. This site guided them so that they could become foster parents. In the back of their minds, they were excited about possibly adopting a child or sibling pair from among the children that they fostered.

No matter what state you live in, enter the name of your state plus the word adoption in your search engine. In some states you can even view photos and profiles of available children arranged according to their age, race or sex. You are doing a beautiful thing to consider fostering and/or adopting a needy child. The biggest shortage is for infants. Older children also need loving parents.

Private Domestic Adoption costs vary from adoption to adoption and state to state. An agency fee ranges from **$15,000 – $30,000.** (https://adoptionnetwork.com › cost-of-adoption › how-much-does-it-cost-to-adopt-a-child)

The average cost range for **International Adoptions** is **$20,000-$40,000** and is a collection of the different expenses that come up over the course of the adoption, including documentation, travel fees, program fees, and more (https://consideringadoption.com › adopting › international-adoption-costs).

In recent years, countries have been less willing to let Americans adopt their orphan children. It seems that people look down on a country which can't place needy children in the homes of its citizens. Historically speaking, the times when it was the easiest to adopt a child from overseas were the years immediately following World Wars I and II.

I deliberately put the following statistic out of place. Think of it as **one more nail in the coffin of the pro-choice myth that abortion is good for all involved.** Study this statistic, you who are undecided about pulling the plug on the life of your unborn child. One of the reasons women submit to having an abortion is that they hope it will save the relationship with their partner. Researcher Emily Milling "found that **of more than 400 cases where unmarried couples had an abortion, 70% split up within a month after the procedure."**

I have followed the work of **Lutherans for Life** for 30 years and I have great respect for their ministry. Roman Catholic **Priests For Life** are especially magnificent pro-life leaders. So are **Anglicans for Life**.

I heartily endorse the **Jewish Pro-life Foundation.** You have suffered a holocaust in the past. May Israel grow in numbers and end abortion. This will eliminate the medical issues abortion causes. You need a swiftly growing population and prosperity in every area, starting with the spiritual realm. May our Jewish friends all become pro-life. May people from all religious and ethnic backgrounds study the advantages of being pro-life and join our cause. Please refer to these ministries in the resource section.

WHY SOME CHILDREN GET STUCK IN FOSTER CARE AND AREN'T MADE AVAILABLE TO BE SWIFTLY ADOPTED AFTER BIRTH

Dr. & Mrs. J.C. Willke explain this in their terrific book, ABORTION, QUESTIONS AND ANSWERS (p.300).

"Actually there are enough couples waiting to adopt minority race babies. But sadly, sometimes they are not adopted. Reasons include the unwillingness of the natural mother to release the child, unwillingness of agencies to allow white parents to adopt them, unrealistically high standards for minority parents to meet in order to qualify, and one more reason, which if true, is a national disgrace. If a baby is placed for adoption at birth, the agency gets X number of dollars. For every child that is in foster care for a year, the agency gets 3X or 4X dollars. The charge has been made that minority race babies are not being placed at birth because the agency needs the additional money it gets for foster care. The system has evolved into an industry with perverse incentives for social agencies to maintain children in the system because of the increased revenue. Some 70% of the money for foster care is spent for administrative overhead and services. **What we have done according to the National Council of Family and Juvenile Court Judges is to 'replace parental neglect with governmental neglect.'"** (R. Woodson, Bureaucratic Barriers to Black Adoption, WALL STREET JOURNAL, June 26, 1984, p.34) (Another problem which prevents the courts from freeing up a child to be adopted is that they are hesitant to declare a mother to be unfit to parent her birth child. **In my opinion, instead of agencies getting incentives for keeping a child in foster care for an extended length of time, they should get bonuses for placing them in permanent homes swiftly.** The faster the babies are adopted, the more the agency should earn. Furthermore, if the couple who adopts the differently-abled child takes the child home from the hospital immediately after birth there is a greater chance that permanent bonding will occur.) The older a differently-abled child becomes, the harder it is to place the child with an adopting family. Foster families should not be required to have separate bedrooms for each child.

MAY WE ALWAYS BE CONSISTENT

I myself have never knowingly voted for a pro-choice candidate. I am a registered Republican. But when the Republicans put a pro-choice candidate, Arnie Carlson, up for governor of Minnesota, I voted for Rudy Perpich, a pro-life Democratic candidate. I think all clergy should refuse to serve communion to candidates who advocate abortion. This is especially true during campaign season when candidates tour trying to get votes and make a point to show up in a church where communion is being served. Let the pastors both refuse to give them communion and give their reasons to the press who are covering the candidates' campaign that day. **I see pro-choice candidates publicaly going to a place of worship in order to fool the voters about their having a strong biblically based life of faith. The fact that these candidates are two faced ought to make all of us angry.**

Had all pro-life citizens refused to vote pro-choice, we could have more swiftly amended our constitution and reversed Roe. But my pro-life friends, take heart. We only need to get enough of them to become consistently pro-life so that we become the clear undisputed majority. Pro-choice voters are killing their own children. They are derailing their own trains (see the poem **"Simple Mathematics"** in Part II Life Triumphs!). **We who love life will therefore absolutely become the majority because our children are turning 18 and voting for life. One of the voting blocs who will help put us over the top are our new citizens and friends entering the United States from Mexico. They are mostly Roman Catholic and pro-life.** Democrats think that by offering welfare benefits to this voting bloc, they can always count on getting the Hispanic vote. But *increasingly our Hispanic friends are going on record to say that it is more important to vote for life than for the bundle of benefits and bribes the pro-choice Democrats hold up in front of them!*

An interesting statistic happened in America in 2019. *Blacks are no longer the largest minority group. Blacks have been systematically brainwashed into aborting their babies. Hispanic-Americans are wiser.* They let their infants live. The trend in America is transforming us into a pro-life and pro-family nation. Gloria A Dios! Glory to God!

TRAGIC NEW YORK MOMENT – CELEBRATION IN KENTUCKY

I think what has happened during the summer of 2019 in New York by Mayor Bill de Blasio is atrocious. *If an abortion fails and the child is born alive, their liberalized laws are deathly cruel. The physician can ask the mother what she wants to happen to the living aborted child. If the mother wishes, she can tell the physician to kill her living child. There is no legal penalty.* In Minnesota, one woman who was a candidate for a late term abortion asked the two doctors who were caring for her what they would do if the child she asked be aborted were born alive. She was stunned to hear they said, "We would break the child's neck." (i.e. kill him or her.)

I believe anyone who supports or votes for a pro-choice candidate or spends money at a pro-choice business is facilitating the murder of innocent children. I define a pro-choice business as one who contributes to abortion facilitators such as Planned Parenthood. *Lists of such stores should be assembled and distributed. It is time to put in place a complete boycott of pro-choice stores.* Our votes and business matter. I believe that boycotting businesses for supporting abortion facilitators such as Planned Parenthood would succeed in getting them to stop funding these abortionists.

Pro-choice advocates in Kentucky encouraged the Supreme Court to hear their protest about two current laws in Kentucky. **Before getting an abortion women must be shown the ultrasound scans of their unborn child and listen to his or her heartbeat.** The Supreme Court refused to hear their case. On December 10, 2019 **the Supreme Court wisely and humanely upheld the law in Kentucky. Pro-life advocates universally recommend that each state insist there be at least a one day delay between when a woman enters an abortion facility and having the procedure.** She also needs to be shown the medical dangers of submitting to an abortion and the benefits of giving a baby up for adoption. Hopefully my idea of compensating both the mother ($2,500) and the person or clinic that encourages her to let her child be adopted ($600) will be put in place ASAP (these fees are open to discussion).

I SUPPORT ABORTION TO PROTECT THE PHYSICAL LIFE OF THE MOTHER

I have a friend who was serving as a Christian missionary in an Arab nation. She was raped. She conceived and never considered aborting her child. The woman and child are beautiful. A fortunate guy won their hearts. She has a terrific marriage. I used to think there were not enough votes to overturn Roe unless we made exceptions for rape, serious birth defects and incest. Thankfully Roe is history! I am enthusiastic about passing nationwide laws to gradually lower the maximum fetal age at which mothers can abort their children. The initial target would be to outlaw all abortions after the child is 19 weeks old (see also p.129), because children who were born at that age have survived. And as far as letting handicapped children be aborted, I wish to tell you about another single friend. She is a prosperous business owner and single parent. She had a blind and autistic baby boy. They are doing great. I know a couple from Canada whose daughter felt she should adopt a Chinese baby with Down's syndrome. She grew older and married later in life so conceiving a child of her own would be difficult. Then she and her husband heard about and adopted a Chinese baby who fit their criteria. They are serving the Lord with YWAM in Canada. Her whole family is totally on board with their loving decision. Her child is a celebrity! **I don't have present knowledge about any children who are born because of an incestuous relationship. But I did help Wendy Simon write her life story, GOOD MOURNING, "one woman's journey from incest and violence to forgiveness, healing and joy."** The difficulties of surviving an incestuous childhood can be overcome. Being introduced to faith in the Lord was the key to her healing. Fortunately, Wendy did not conceive a child. I will always support abortion if it is necessary to protect the physical life of the mother.

Former abortionist Doctor Anthony Levatino whom we've already discussed earlier in this book is also an attorney. He explains that legalizing abortion for the health of the mother is too broad. It could refer to the financial health, the social health, the emotional health, etc. He believes it is just fine to support legislation if to have the baby would jeopardize the physical life of the mother. **As a former abortionist who completed 1,200 procedures, he never once encountered a woman who needed an abortion to save her life.** I agree with him. I most certainly do not support abortion for sex selection. But *I favor supporting expectant mothers who fall into these four categories by helping them in practical and emotional ways so they can go forward with their pregnancies.* Some expectant mothers have been told their child may be seriously handicapped. If they don't wish to raise their child they should check the resource section to see if any family might like to adopt their differently-abled child. The shortage of infants available to be adopted makes this increasingly likely. **Hopefully women in these categories won't wait until a law forces them to carry their crisis pregnancy to term. May these women study the arguments for life and risks of abortion and make a wise loving choice without compulsion! May they own their decision. May these honorable women and the father of their child each have someone stand with them.**

Bob and Pam were missionaries in the Philippines. Pam became pregnant. Unfortunately she caught a life threatening disease, amoebic dysentery. Her doctor said, "If you want to live, the baby will have to die." Pam refused an abortion. She risked her life for the sake of their unborn child. That child was Tim Tebow, Heisman Trophy winner sportscaster and professional baseball player, recently married to Miss Universe. (https://timtebow.com/)

~~To summarize at this time I support these exemptions. Allowing these exceptions is the most efficient and fastest way to lower the number of abortions in America.~~

A PREGNANT WOMAN'S MOST IMPORTANT NEED

What is the most devastating single statistic as we consider the problem of defeating abortion? In one survey of women in crisis pregnancies who aborted, *more than half said they would have given birth if someone, the father, ANYONE would have said, "I will be here for you."* Reread these words out loud three times. Memorize them. Celebrate the power of encouragement. Someday the unborn child will thank you. The mother will thank you now. Locate the father and encourage him if he is not standing up for his child, to be a man rather than a wimp. This is the only way fathers can be respected. All parents in a crisis pregnancy situation need consistent support. Be pleasantly assertive and offer verbal and practical encouragement liberally.

THE MOST DIFFICULT EXPERIENCE OF MY LIFE

I am directing these next words to you gentlemen. Please, **please do not plan on having unlimited time to express your love to your woman.** When my wife was 27 and our son was six months old, tragedy struck. The previous weekend I had taken her to Palm Springs, California. I went all out to love and appreciate my wife and our son. We had a wonderful vacation. Driving home to San Bernardino she said, "This is the best weekend we have ever had!" I agreed. She was having an unusually severe headache.

Four days later, my wife called me at work. She said she thought she had experienced a seizure. She explained she had been holding our son in the rocking chair. She awoke sixty minutes later, lying on the sofa still holding him. Fortunately she did not drop him. She had thrown up. I took her into the ER where they examined her. They were not convinced it was a seizure. They sent her home with instructions to rest. Early Saturday morning, she woke me up while having a grand mall seizure. John and Penny lived across the hall in our apartment. Penny watched our son.

John and I admitted her to the hospital. She had a series of seizures. She would sleep following each one...then awaken for a short time. Each time she was less and less alert. My mom flew in from Minneapolis that evening. Sunday morning I was with my wife in the hospital. She sent me home to get her nursing bra. Her breasts were engorged. I also brought her a get well card. She could not open it. I did and asked her to read it. She could not. So I asked how it was signed. She said, "Love always." Those were the last words she would ever speak. She never woke up again. Monday morning one of her anesthetist colleagues, Doug Nielson, came to visit her. My wife and I were Godparents to his and Yuki's young daughter. I was telling Doug what a wonderful wife she was to me and mom she was to our son, and her eyes teared up. I am convinced she could hear my words. I walked Doug to his car. When I reentered the hospital, the loudspeaker urgently announced, "Code Blue 3 East!" My wife had coded. They got her heart started and put her on a respirator. Her neurologist inserted dye into her body and took an X-ray to see what was going on. He said, "I'm sorry, Dale, but her brain has swollen. I could not get any dye into it. You should gather your family around you." She died the next day just an hour after her mom came from Felton, MN to visit her. Grandma Emma Olek brought my son home with her on the plane. My mom and I drove.

My in-laws requested the memorial service be held in Northern Minnesota in their home church in Felton. That afternoon my parents thankfully invited my son and me to rent from them. What a Godsend! I flew back to resign my job, sell our furniture, close up our home and pack up what I could in a small travel trailer to bring to Fridley, MN, a suburb of Minneapolis. Beyond any doubt, that first night I spent in the apartment was the loneliest of my entire life. That evening the Lord gave me this Christmas carol, MESSIAH IN A MANGER. It expresses the Messiah's stepfather Joseph's joyful point of view. Hours earlier, he supported his wife Mary as she birthed the Messiah. My dear brothers, follow Joseph's lead. **No one needs love and support more than a new mother!** I encourage you to be the very, very best hero to the mother and your growing child. They need you and expect you to do the right thing by them.

MESSIAH IN A MANGER

Advent prepares the world for Jesus' birth.
Prophets of old foretell God's trip to earth…
Why would God let His only Son come down
    leaving the golden streets for Beth'lem town?

Jesus came down, was a little baby.
Wise men thought that maybe
    He would rule the world with love,
    compassion, understanding,
    happiness and peace forever more.

Frost filled the air. Angelic melodies.
Look now, young Joseph holds Christ on his knees.
Jesus' small hand gives father's beard a tug.
The laughing Joseph gives his son a hug.

Mary watches. Overwhelming gladness!
Gone are birth pangs, sadness.
Every evil vanishes.
Tonight she has a man child.
Happiness and peace for ever more.

High on the hills there is a small campfire.
Suddenly shepherds hear an angel choir!
Bright lights at night give shepherds chills and fear.
"Be not afraid, because Emmanuel's here!"

Shepherd's running down the hills together.
Who cares if the weather's freezing cold?
The Lord is born! Messiah in a manger!
Happiness and peace for ever more.

Shepherd's gone…The virgin lies a sleeping.
Joseph softly weeping. Tears of joy
    fall down and kiss the Infant Jesus' fingers.
Happiness and peace for ever more.

Happiness for you! Peace! Ever more!

THE LUTHERAN AMBASSADOR, December 1972,
used by permission

JOIN THE LIFE VOTERS ALLIANCE (LVA)

Those who join would do three things (Our platform consists of sixteen words):

    Only vote for pro-life candidates
    Only vote for a pro-life party
    Only shop at pro-life businesses

I just coined the phrase **Life Voters' Alliance**. This organization will donate copies of CHOOSE LIFE to people who are entering pro-choice and pro-life counseling centers. We welcome anyone who would like to fund these gifts to join us. I am pleased to endorse and help candidates from any party who share my views. Please join our mailing list.

Right now even though they are pro-life at heart, because they have always voted Democratic in the past, some pro-life Democrats unwisely continue to support Democratic candidates. We need to educate and encourage our Democratic friends to be consistent. They see other aspects of the Democratic platform which appeal to them. **These Democrats have yet to believe that they should never compromise on the issue of life.** The seven last words for these Democrats are, "We've always done it this way before." We who are against abortion need to wisely reach out, educate and invite them to stand with us and against abortion. (Use the statistics in this document to educate our pro-choice friends. Our friends need us to be proactive.)

HOW IS SEX SELECTION ABORTION HARMING OUR FRIENDS IN CHINA?

China has been limiting couples to having only one child. Tradition in China designates the oldest son as being the one to care for his aging parents. This is the main reason why the Chinese aborted more female infants. "The solution to China's demographic time bomb lies in changing age-old attitudes." As of May, 2021, our most important trading partner and friends in China now officially allow some couples to have three children.

They still have 30 million more Chinese men than women, but this wise policy will gradually right itself. Plus by improving the ratio of wage earners to retirees, their economy will improve. (Source: https://www.scmp.com › News › China › Politics)

DOES A MOTHER FEEL PAIN DURING AN ABORTION?

On the abort73.com website, 771 women reported that they regretted having the abortion. But 39 women reported they were glad they had the procedure. The following case studies you will now read indicate, they had some negative feelings about the difficulty they experienced during the procedure. These case studies were voluntarily emailed to abort73.com. I encourage you to read some more of them.

One woman said she, "wouldn't wish a surgical or medical abortion on her worst enemy." Many spoke of horrific debilitating pain as evidenced by the excerpts below:

"Toward the end of the procedure, it became excruciatingly painful. I have multiple huge tattoos, but I have NEVER felt pain like that before…it was burning and agonizing." (24-year old woman from Atlanta)

"I had no idea it would be this bad. I was writhing in pain. I couldn't stay still. I was shivering with cold. The abortion went on for 1.5 hours. Then the bleeding began. I took another pain killer…but, I was unable to take the pain." (22-year old woman from India)

"It was the most intense pain I have ever felt in my life. Never in my wildest dreams did I think I would ever have to feel this amount of pain…it was pure torture. I kept saying, 'I can't handle this,' as my cervix became more and more dilated. The pain was unbelievable…my brain just kept saying, 'Get out of there! Stop what you are doing!!' It was roughly 10 minutes of pain equal to all my bones breaking." (23-year old woman from Pennsylvania)

"I got the abortion at Planned Parenthood after I had been pregnant for 8 weeks. I took 800 mg Ibuprofen and two Vicodin pills that I was offered. The stretching of the cervix was excruciating and actually made me vomit." (21-year old woman)

"About 20 minutes in I noticed light cramps and knew I was in for some hard pain. I took another codeine even though I hadn't completely dissolved the chalky abortion pills sitting in my mouth. From here, the pain intensified one thousand fold. I would feel waves of it rushing through my belly, tightening and throbbing similar to period pain, but with an added dose of raw, relentless PAIN." (19-year old woman from Australia)

Another 67-year old woman from Canada wrote, "In the years following my abortion, there was this deep pain in my chest. It was always there and it felt as though someone had plunged a knife in my heart and I longed for someone to just pull it out!"

THE PHYSICAL LIFE OF THE MOTHER ALWAYS COMES FIRST

On one principle, I do not compromise. The physical health and life of the mother always comes first! This is the main reason why I am so incensed at the financially greedy abortion industry. **They hide the dangers to mothers.** A generation of victims of abortion have been mutilated, rendered sterile and instead of having gorgeous enchanting enlarged breasts (this happens when a mother nurses her child) and celebrating the privilege of nursing healthy infants, many lost their breasts to an elective disease, "breast cancer caused by abortion." As part of the physical the mother gets before having an abortion, I suggest having the doctor take topless photos of her from the front and from each side from the waist up. The photos would be placed safely in her medical records and she would keep copies. (Medical records are presently spotty at best. Each woman deserves to have a permanent file documenting her abortion.) Then if she gets breast cancer should she desire to litigate against the abortion facility that promised her a safe abortion, the jury can see how she was cruelly disfigured. Is it fair that pro-choice business people urge women to abort what may be the only child they can ever conceive?

America is increasingly becoming pro-life. A Gallup poll taken May 18, 2018 reported **pro-life and pro-choice voters are tied at 48%. The remaining folks are undecided, waiting for us to educate and encourage them.** My warmest greetings to our undecided friends and future allies for life!!

WURMBRAND'S VISION - YOUR VISION

When Richard and Sabina Wurmbrand first married and they conceived a child, they had an abortion. They preferred to not interrupt their life of pleasure with the inconvenience of a baby. Then a simple retired carpenter prayed, "God I know I will get my reward in heaven. But I would like it now. I would like to help a Jewish person believe in you. There are no Jews in my small town. I don't have funds to travel. So, it is up to you to bring me a Jew." When the Wurmbrands arrived he courted Richard like a suitor would an irresistibly lovely potential wife. He described God's love and gave him a Bible. One day Wurmbrand was lying on his sofa reading it with his long legs sticking over the armrest. He wished to understand it, but failed to. So he prayed, "God, I am small and you are big. So it is Your job to find me, not mine to find You." Then he laid the open Bible on his chest and waited. Moments later, Jesus appeared to Wurmbrand in a vision. As a result, he soon became a strong believer. He also developed as a leader in the underground church boldly resisting atheistic communism. Rumania would go on to vote him one of the ten most influential Rumanian citizens of all time.

You are probably wondering how becoming a believer affected Wurmbrand's attitude towards having children. They first had their own son, Michael. Then as WWII progressed, they adopted six Jewish orphans. When an opportunity came to put them on a ship to Israel, they did so. Unfortunately, Nazi submarines sunk the boat and the children all perished.

Following 14 years spent in communist prisons, his family was ransomed from communist Rumania to the west for $10,000 by Norwegian Christians. He developed a ministry to help persecuted Christians and Jews. His son Michael continues reaching out to families who have suffered under communism. You may get Wurmbrand's complimentary newsletter by emailing mw@helpforreffugees.com. Wurmbrand wrote TORTURED FOR CHRIST and CHRIST ON THE JEWISH ROAD. Other of his titles are listed on amazon.com. A free copy of TORTURED FOR CHRIST and their newsletter are available upon request.

Not long ago I read JESUS VISIONS, MIRACLES AMONG MOSLEMS, by Christine Darg (https://jerusalemchannel.tv/exploits-magazine/). She alleges that **25% of our Moslem friends who become believers are singled out by the Lord who comes to them in a vision**. The case studies are amazing. You may get a complimentary subscription to her monthly magazine by writing exploitsministries@mac.com. Buy JESUS VISIONS. If you wish, you can tell the Lord you are open to getting a vision of Him. For sure do what Wurmbrand did and read the Bible. Call the folks in the enclosed RESOURCE SECTION.

I suggest you research Richard Wurmbrand's name on the internet and learn more. When my beloved wife died at age 27, I was working full time for Wurmbrand. That someone makes a mistake on the abortion issue does not end one's life. I urge you to listen to one or two of his sermons which are posted on the internet.

MY MOM'S FRIEND

My mom had a wonderful friend who basically checked out and disappeared for some months not long after they finished high school. Mom said she was vague about what was going on in her life. Because she was exceptionally pretty and gifted, mom said she was surprised she never married. Fast forward. When mom was in her late forties, this friend called her and excitedly said, "My son contacted me! He is a pastor!"

Then her friend explained that the reason she was away from town for some months long ago was because she had been raped. She conceived a son, was embarrassed, moved away, birthed him, and then put him up for adoption. And that her son had sought her out, wondering about the circumstances which led to her giving him away. Her son welcomed her into his life and proudly introduced her to his wife and her grandchildren. It turns out her son inherited her musical gifts. They went on to sing duets together. She also explained that the reason she never married was because she felt she was damaged goods, and that no one would want her. What is the takeaway from this fabulous true story? **Even if the circumstances surrounding your conceiving a child were not ideal, if you ask, the Lord can bring you through it**. Selectively share your challenges with key people in your life. God gives us direction and encouragement.

If this book influenced you to birth your child, I would also love to see an ultrasound or a photo of your child. Please enclose your contact information. **You are welcome to share what in this book helped you**. If I may have permission to quote your comments and use the photo of your child, that would also be appreciated. I believe that readers who see subsequent editions of this book would be encouraged to birth their child if they saw photos of children whose mothers decided to CHOOSE LIFE.

I hope to find funds so this book may be printed and made available, for example, to give freely to people who are entering both pro-life and pro-choice crisis pregnancy facilities. May my words prevent needy mothers from being harmed by abortionists. Instead may they keep their unborn children or offer them up to those qualified loving couples and individuals who are seeking to have a child. **Let's unite to support those in crisis pregnancy situations and love their unborn infants**. Please study information about the ministries in the reference section. Interact with and support them.

IF YOU HAD AN ABORTION, YOUR CHILD IS IN HEAVEN WITH JESUS – WHAT DO YOU LONG TO TELL YOUR UNBORN CHILD?

I think that one advantage of committing your life to Jesus and believing in and living for Him is that you will eventually be able to meet your unborn child in heaven. You may write the first words you will speak to your child in your heart now. And keep them in your mind. Be sure your relationship with God is in good repair. Read the four gospels and study the life of Jesus. Ask Jesus to strengthen your faith in Him and for help to make choices which will honor Him and your strong growing family.

MY CONCLUDING THOUGHTS

Please, everyone, join me and step back from what has happened and look at our beloved country.

Roe vs. Wade would never have passed if honest statistics had been used regarding how many mothers lost their lives through illegal abortion.

There exists for every nation an optimum ratio of people working and people who are retired. Let the authorities in America discover what this ratio is and devise a way repair it.

The single most logical way to repair the ratio is to increase the number of children being born each year. Although it will take time we need to start on it right away.

Where else can our nation get help to repair the ratio? America is blessed because we have immigrants willing to move to America and work to build successful lives and families. I myself am a second generation American. My mom's father was from Oslo, Norway where he was working in the palace as a jewelry designer for the king. My dad's father was born on a large dairy farm near Copenhagen, Denmark. Of all the various sectors in America who have learned to use immigrant labor, agriculture is the most successful. Individual farmers wisely make specific requests for people they need and when they will need them.

But what should America do now? I want to motivate all parties to discover and do God's will for them. I recommend the following changes:

Those working in the abortion industry - such as Dr. Levatino to become a force for good, standing up for life. I'm happy to report that some abortion clinics are closing because they can't find staff willing to abort children.

Those deciding if they should let their child live or take their unborn child's life – to celebrate and support life.

For abortion facilities to become pro-life as I have explained in this book, increasing their incomes and getting God's blessings.

Those harmed by abortion - to turn to the Lord for forgiveness and to draw on his strength to make the wisest choices as they look to the future.

Legislators - to rewrite laws so God is honored and Satan, the angel of death is identified and put in his place - may Satan's plans be systematically revealed, reversed and defeated.

To reward counselors and agencies who sign up couples to put their child up for adoption with $600.

To reward mothers in crisis pregnancies who give their child up for adoption to get $2,500. (These sums are open for discussion.) These funds will be paid by those adopting the child.

Our nation - that we can unite and repent creating a safe haven where all unborn children can be born, be supported, and not just accepted, but celebrated.

Our economy – we must correct the imbalance between workers and retirees. We need to selectively encourage and recruit immigrants whose work skills will help America prosper. The two most important things which keep someone from living in poverty are: 1) to get married before having their first child, 2) to finish high school or earn a GED.

Those who finish high school have greater lifetime earnings. In order to keep teenagers from dropping out of school, (this only affects families receiving welfare and food stamps) we should require teenagers to stay in school, have no more than one unexcused absence per month and maintain a

C average. Working on a GED would also be acceptable. If the teenager cannot do that, the family will not get any welfare benefits for the teenager. (Therefore if the teenager has dropped out of high school he or she will be given 30 days to reenroll in high school or sign up to get a GED. If we let a teenager drop out of school as many of them do, and they don't get a job, we are programming them to be losers. Ideally they will treat going to school as if it were a job which pays them and their family their welfare and food stamp benefits. I believe the school counselors should give students returning to school the option of getting high school credit for working an appropriate paying part time job. This would give positive reinforcement for them to be successful to complete their high school degree or GED.)
It would be to America's advantage to prioritize inviting immigrants with many children or who plan to raise large families. If we wisely analyze the job openings we have today and the ones we will have in the future, our education system can train the appropriate number of workers we will need to make our economy thrive. Therefore, a key benefit of outlawing abortion is that we will increasingly have enough workers born by healthy mothers generating enough income to put America's budget in the black and reduce the national debt.

Although I am not with you in person, I hope you can sense my friendship and love flowing through my fingertips and computer to bless you. Please join me in praying that the power of God's love will soften and transform the hearts of all who are in the abortion industry. **May they only use their skills to heal and give life.** I have outlined a way they could increase their corporate profits and remove the barriers between them and God.

HOW I BEGIN MY DAY – HOW I TOOK THE TITLE POET-PHILOSOPHER

A certain pastor of a prominent large church in NYC noticed a blue collar person would go up to the altar and kneel reverently for a moment during his lunch hour, then depart.

One day he stopped the man as he was leaving, introduced himself, smiled and said, "You are most welcome in our church. Thanks for coming. May I ask what you pray when you use part of your lunch hour to come into our church?" The man smiled and said, "I just pray, God it's me Jimmy. I want Him to know I am recognizing Him and thankful that He is in my life." It was perhaps a decade ago that I began to daily follow the example of this blue collar working man. I am blessed with a lake home. And I go to the lake shore early each day. I rest my right hand on the wall of the fire pit, and I lightly touch my right knee to a board on the ground. Then I pray 12 words, **"Dear God, it's me, Dale and I long to do Your will."** Then I stand and add more specific prayer requests. I keep a path from my split entry home to the lake shoveled all winter so I can pay my respects to the Lord. It is my way of giving myself totally to the Lord. I have one of those Olympic style racing boats with a sliding seat. Most warm days I will then go out for a row or sit in a lawn chair reading a portion from the Bible or a Christian book. *"Faith comes by hearing and hearing by the word of God"* (Romans 10:17). I sold my lake home, but I continue praying in this manner outside my new home.

Thank you for soldiering through my poems and thoughts. You may contact me through the publisher or through my email at choose1life@outlook.com. If you wish to share a brief comment about how this book has encouraged you to CHOOSE LIFE and you permit me to use your comments and possibly the photo of your child in order to publicize future editions of my book or my CHOOSE LIFE book blog, I would greatly appreciate it.

I would like to thank my friend and author, Pastor **Dennis Gray**, owner of Mercy and Truth Publishers in Argyle, MN for encouraging me to write this book. I also thank the people who have had an abortion or adoption experience and those who formerly worked in the abortion industry or interacted with abortion providers for their key contributions. I also want to thank **Laura Peterson** and **Linda Lopez** from Lakeside Press for their cover design and page layout and my editor, **Carol Lenhart**.

Italo Calvino penned these words, "Were I to choose an auspicious image for the new millennium, I would choose this one: the sudden agile leap of the **poet-philosopher** who raises himself above the weight of the world, showing that with all its gravity he has the secret of lightness, and that what many consider to be the vitality of the times–noise, aggressive, revving and roaring–belongs to the realm of death, like a cemetery for rusty old cars."

I invite pro-choice advocates to send me their poems.

RESOURCE CENTER

AARP: The American Association of Retired People
866-654-5572
https://www.aarp.org/
It is to the advantage of retired people to have as many people working as possible, so we encourage AARP to be pro-life.

Abortion Procedures:
https://www.abortionprocedures.com/

ABORTION'S SECOND VICTIM: (Pam Koerbel's story describing how she became pregnant, rationalized aborting her child and found "forgiveness and emotional healing")

Abortion Risks:
Louisiana and Texas Department of State Health Services
225-342-9500
512-834-6628
http://ldh.la.gov/
https://www.dshs.state.tx.us/

Abort73.com:
https://abort73.com/
They focus on ministry to high school and college students. Describes the Potential for Abortion Clinic Abuse. Aborting women are vulnerable to the predatory behavior of unscrupulous doctors. **This informative site contains 771 unsolicited abortion stories and details about Post Abortion Syndrome**. The website for the largest abortion provider in America, Planned Parenthood, has this to say about the risks of abortion, **"Abortion does not cause breast cancer. Safe, uncomplicated abortion does not cause problems for future pregnancies such as birth defects, premature birth or low birth weight babies, ectopic pregnancy, miscarriage, or infant death."** Abort73.com gives convincing evidence that these claims are false. The mortality rate for example of women who get breast cancer is 20%. **Set aside a block of time and study abort73. com together with the representative from your abortion**

provider. **Get involved.** Abortion persists because of our ignorance, apathy and confusion. This site also contains excellent descriptions of the various types of abortion. They also have an encouraging section which will help people who have already had an abortion.

Adult & Teen Challenge USA:
417-581-2181
info@teenchallengeusa.org/
5250 N Towne Center Drive
Ozark, MO 65721
They treat drug and alcohol dependencies. When people with dependencies are selecting a treatment program, they should know that faith-based treatment programs are more successful than secular ones. Get founder Dave Wilkerson's book or movie "THE CROSS AND THE SWITCHBLADE."

Alcohol Abuse: Al-Anon Family Groups:
800-356-9996
757-563-1600
https://al-anon.org/
Al-Anon is a branch of Alcoholics Anonymous.

Alcoholics Victorious:
https://www.alcoholicsvictorious.org/database/
They were founded as a Christian alternative to Alcoholics Anonymous. When AA starts their meetings people introduce themselves by their first names and they say, "My name is … and I am an alcoholic." AA teaches once you're an alcoholic, you're always an alcoholic. When they bury you, they bury a dead alcoholic. The theme verse for AV is, *"Any man is in Christ, he is a new creature. Old things have passed away and all things have become new"* (2 Corinthians 5:17).
The Alcoholics Victorious Creed:
I realize that I cannot overcome my addiction by myself. I believe that the power of Jesus Christ is available to help me. I believe that through my acceptance of Him as my Savior, I am a new person. Because the presence of God is manifested through continued prayer, I will set aside two periods every day, morning and evening, for communion with

my Heavenly father. I realize my need for daily Bible reading and use it as a guide for my daily living. (Psalm 27:11-15) I recognize my need of Christian fellowship and will, therefore, have fellowship with Christians through the church of my choice. I know that in order to be victorious, I must keep active in the service of Christ and His Church and I will help others to victory. (Hebrews 10:23-25) I do not partake of any beverage containing alcohol. I know it is the first drink that does the harm. Therefore, "I do not drink." I can be victorious because I know that God's strength is sufficient to supply all my needs. (Philippians 4:19)

American Association of Pro-Life Obstetricians and Gynecologists (AAPLOG):
443-640-1051
https://www.aaogf.org/
2331 Rock Spring Rd.
Forest Hill, MD 21050
tim@stringfellowgroup.net

American Pregnancy Association:
800-672-2296
https://americanpregnancy.org/
Knowledge is power. They are a gold mine of information during the whole chronological process of becoming pregnant: overcoming infertility, which nutrients to take to prevent miscarriage and birth defects, a weekly update for the mother as her baby grows and describes the details and dangers of abortion, finding a group home where a woman may live during her pregnancy, adoption options including financial help, baby names, etc. Treat yourself to their encouraging web site! They permit a mother to follow her pregnancy week-by-week. Some of what I will share comes from their website. **They can direct you to help, including abortion alternatives near you. Simply share your zip code with them.** Some abortion clinics perform abortions on young girls without requiring them to identify the father. In some cases, the father was a family member. Should these men be permitted to go unpunished?

Anglicans for Life
412-749-0455
https://anglicansforlife.org/
President Georgette Fornay also co-founded Silent No More ministry.

Association of Mature American Citizens (AMAC):
888-262-2006
https://amac.us/
These folks are pro-life. They are the conservative alternative to AARP.

Bethany Christian Services:
800-BETHANY
https://bethany.org/

Carenet:
715-532-7600
800-518-7909
https://www.care-net.org/
CareNet is a comprehensive pro-life ministry. Their Pregnancy Decision Line does free real-time pregnancy coaching to parents making life and death decisions about their babies. They have a network of 1,100 affiliated pregnancy centers ministering in person to all who come in. They have church partners who train their congregations to offer compassion, hope and help to anyone considering abortion. (Perhaps your church or synagogue could join them?) **They have free online courses which have trained 30,000 people to intercede for lives at risk. From 2008 to January 2020 Carenet's pro-life team recorded that 708,686 preborn lives were saved through their ministry. All are welcome to call.**

Catholic Charities:
https://www.catholiccharitiesusa.org/
Dioceses throughout the country provide adoption assistance.

Comprehensive Sex Ed (CSE):
On April 23, 2019 the majority of State Representatives in the Minnesota House tragically voted to mandate (H.F.1414) every Pre K-12 public/charter school to teach "Comprehensive Sex Ed (CSE). CSE removes all natural and

protective boundaries for children and teens, encouraging sexual exploration in graphic detail. CSE uses borderline pornographic illustrations and graphic descriptions to teach children as young as 10 that all "consensual" sexual activity is their "right". The CSE people encourage the youth to exclude their parents from learning about what they are being taught. CSE allows unlicensed Planned Parenthood and gender identity activists into your child's classroom to teach these dangerous and unhealthy practices. CSE actually grooms children for early sexual activity making them vulnerable targets for sexual abuse, experimentation and trafficking.

CSE is also dangerous because it encourages random sexual encounters. Web MD says, "It can take 3-12 weeks for the AIDS virus to show up on routine tests for the infection which measures antibodies against HIV. Therefore a person can carry the AIDS virus without knowing they are contagious. CSE overemphasizes the physical aspects of sexuality to the narrow confines of the genitals. They prematurely sexualize youth. Song of Solomon 2:7, 3:5 and 8:4 warns us, *"Do not stir up or awaken love until it pleases."* The ideal place for a man and woman to give themselves fully in a romantic way is in marriage. God's ideal is one man for one woman for one life time. Purity until marriage also eliminates STDs.

In order to expand a couple's relationship with each other, please refer to my poems in Plan A of CHOOSE LIFE.

Child Protection League:
888-538-3188
https://cplaction.com/
PO Box 463
Mankato, MN 56002
The Child Protection League (CPL) is committed to promoting the welfare of children and protecting them from exploitation, indoctrination and violence. They educate citizens on issues that protect or threaten the safety of children. CPL supports the rights of children to:
• Freely express their political beliefs, moral standards, and faith

- Experience personal, physical privacy and modesty in bathrooms, showers, locker rooms, and living spaces separated by biological sex
- Experience safe classrooms with common-sense disciplinary policies
- Personal data privacy
- Have their safety, education, and healthcare protected and directed by their parents
- Receive an education free from political biases and unscientific ideologies

For more details, download their CPL Flyer (PDF). I urge you to get on their mailing list, ask for their information packet and join the fight.

Choose Life America
352-624-2854
http://www.choose-life.org/contact.php
Proceeds from their designer license plates which are available in most states help fund pro-life activities. You may choose to call to request financial help.

Embryo Adoption Program:
615-321-8866
https://embryoadoptionusa.com/embryo-adoption-program/
They encourage people to adopt leftover embryos. There are approximately 1.4 million in storage. 10% are abandoned.

Family Life Services:
800-388-3336
https://familylifeservices.org/

Family Life Today:
Phone: 434-845-5334
Toll-Free Hotline: 855-677-8620
https://www.familylife.com/podcast/familylife-today/
P.O. Box 4199
Lynchburg VA 24502
Family Life Today has an outstanding daily radio show. I encourage you to contact them to find out when it plays in your community.

Focus on the Family:
800-A-FAMILY (232-6459)
https://www.focusonthefamily.com/
8605 Explorer Drive
Colorado Springs, CO 80920-1051
I suggest you call them to find out when their excellent radio program airs in your community. They are a full service family ministry which deals with many of the abortion related issues in CHOOSE LIFE. My grandchildren enjoy their magazines for kids.

Glamcheck:
https://www.glamcheck.com/health/2012/06/r-breast-cancer-how-are-they-related
Valuable information documenting the connection between breast cancer and abortion

Healing Hearts Hotline:
888-217-8679
630-990-0909 (Illinois)
https://www.healinghearts.org/

Healing Hearts Center
800-828-7893
https://www.healing-hearts-center.org/
P.O. Box 3111
Waxahachie, TX 75168
Email: healingheartscenter@yahoo.com

Heartbeat International:
800-712-HELP
https://www.heartbeatinternational.org/
They founded the first network of pro-life pregnancy resource centers in the US and is the most extensive in the world. Since its establishment in 1971, Heartbeat has supported and/or started more than 2,800 pregnancy help locations worldwide to offer women alternatives to abortion. It is a non-profit federation of faith-based pregnancy resource centers, medical clinics, maternity homes and non-profit adoption agencies. **The Option Line is the U.S's only fully-staffed 24/7/365 bilingual pro-life contact center offering**

counseling in English and Spanish. *Gloria A Dios! Glory to God!* *It has reached more than 3.75 million women and men and helped countless more since its establishment in 2003.* Heartbeat's commitment is *"No woman should feel alone, coerced, or so hopeless that she ends her child's life through abortion."* Counselors are committed to care and competence. "No matter where you are in the world, abortion ends the life of a developing human baby, and while different countries have their cultures and varied ways of communicating, the fact remains that abortion carries risks to women." Betty McDowell, Heartbeat International vice president added, "Every woman has a right to know all the information before making an abortion decision. Denying women awareness of the emotional, psychological and physical risks that abortion can cause would be neglectful and dangerous."

Human Life International (HLI):
800-549-5433
https://www.hli.org/
4 Family Life Lane
Front Royal, VA 22630

Jack Hayford Ministries:
800-776-8180
https://www.jackhayford.org/
Author of I'LL HOLD YOU IN HEAVEN

Jesus Film Project:
407-826-2300
https://www.jesusfilm.org/
You may watch the gospel of Luke from the Bible. It has been made into a movie. Go to jesusfilm.org/. Select from 1,700 languages. It is the most widely viewed and translated movie of all time. This film will strengthen your faith, encourage your spirit and bless you. Some people have even been miraculously healed while watching it. The Jesus film is also available in a children's version.

Jewish Pro-Life Foundation:
412-758-3269
https://jewishprolifefoundation.org/

Lila Rose: Live Action:
https://www.liveaction.org/
Founder and President Lila Rose started Live Action when she was just 15 years old from her family's living room. Since that time, Live Action has grown to become one of the leading national pro-life and human rights organizations in America, dedicated to ending abortion and inspiring a culture that respects and defends life. (See part 6 of CHOOSE LIFE, abortion workers and picketers, where she interviews former abortionist Dr. Anthony Levatino.)

Lutherans For Life:
888-21-STORY
https://www.lutheransforlife.org/
Email: information@lutheransforlife.org
1120 South G Avenue, Nevada, IA 50201)
For Bible based and gospel focused materials on abortion, adoption **including placing differently-abled children**, bioethics, creation, end-of-life, family living, fetal development, sexual purity and post abortion healing. One of my goals in writing this brochure is to fulfill James 4:22. *"Do not merrily listen to the word, and so deceive yourself. Do what it says."* Lutherans For Life has a terrific free educational packet. They even have church bulletin inserts.

McDowell, Josh and Sean:
Josh McDowell Ministry
866-252-5424
https://www.josh.org/
Authors of MORE THAN A CARPENTER by (This is my first recommendation if you want to get a book which will give you an easy to read well documented description of Christianity. Their book called WHY WAIT gives an outstanding presentation about **the advantages of saving oneself for marriage.**)

My Pregnancy Choices Life Care Center:
952-997-2229
https://mypregnancychoices.com/
Becky Hanel, Executive Director
5010 Glazier Ave #104
Apple Valley, MN 55124

National AIDS Hotline:
800-342-AIDS
https://www.ncbi.nlm.nih.gov › pubmed

National Health Information Center:
800-336-4797
https://health.gov/our-work/health-literacy/resources/national-health-information-center

National Right to Life: 202-626-8800
https://www.nrlc.org/outreach/
1446 Duke Street
Alexandria, VA 22314
They are a religious outreach. They have additional programs such as for American Victims of Abortion, Teens for Life, state legislative initiatives, etc.

National Runaway Switchboard: (Runaways)
800-621-4000
https://www.1800runaway.org/

National STD Hotline:
800-227-8922
They help people deal with sexually transmitted diseases. (Pro-choice training materials unfortunately sometimes forget to identify the many STD's which are transmitted by skin to skin contact, even if the man is always correctly wearing a new condom during intercourse.)

Nightlight Christian Adoptions:
502-423-5780
https://www.nightlight.org/snowflakes-embryo-adoption-donation/embryo-adoption/
For those who are unable to successfully conceive a child.

OCTOBER BABY:
https://www.octoberbabymovie.net/
The movie OCTOBER BABY tells the story of Gianna Jessen who survived an abortion.

Open Democracy:
https://www.opendemocracy.net/en/
This liberal group funds pro-choice activities. It advocates abortion and left wing policies through its reporting and analysis of social and political issues. Its fiscal sponsor is NEO Philanthropy, which Capital Research Center's (CRC) is a fiscal clearing house for left-of-center causes. Much of NEO's nearly $340 million in revenues comes from the liberal Ford Foundation and George Soros's foundation to Promote Open Society. They promote women's rights in support of abortion.

THE PASSION OF THE CHRIST by Mel Gibson:
The next most widely viewed film about Jesus' life after JESUSFILM.ORG.

Pharmacists For Life:
740-881-5520
http://www.pfli.org/
P O Box 1281
Powell, OH 43065-1281
The only website serving the profession of pharmacy has a totally 100% pro-life philosophy! All the pro-life pharmacy news and information that is fit to print and that the "drive-by" pharmacy media choose to ignore or misreport. On January 2020 their website reports, "250,000,000 estimated American deaths by chemical abortion since Roe vs. Wade and Doe vs. Bolton."

Pregnancy Center Truth:
Pregnancy Hotline: 800-848-LOVE
https://pregnancycentertruth.com/
Discover general information about pro-life clinics.

PRIDE:
800-241-7946
https://www.pride.com/
Drug Abuse

Priests For Life:
321-500-1000
888-735-3448
https://www.priestsforlife.org/
Email: mail@priestsforlife.org
PO Box 23669 Cocoa, FL 32923
Fr. Frank Pavone, National Director and Chairman of the Board
Janet Morana, Executive Director
They have an amazing powerful and diverse website which
describes excellent groups of programs for clergy and lay
people.

Pro-Life Across America: (The Billboard People)
612-781-0410
800-366-7773
https://prolifeacrossamerica.org/
They average 250 people calling in to discuss crisis
pregnancies each month.

Pro-Life Action Ministries:
651-771-1500
https://plam.org/
Email: prolife@plam.org
1163 Payne Avenue
Saint Paul, MN 55130

Pro-Life Alliance of Gays and Lesbians:
202-223-6697
http://www.plagal.org/
I want to give these **valued allies for life** a special shout out.

Rachel's Vineyard Ministries:
(610) 354-0555
866-482-5433
808 N. Henderson Road 2nd Floor
King of Prussia, PA 19406
https://www.rachelsvineyard.org/
**Rachel's Vineyard is the largest post abortion healing
ministry in the world.** If you had a painful abortion
experience, I strongly urge you to check them out.

Silent No More Awareness: 888-735-3448
https://www.silentnomoreawareness.org/
Email: mail@silentnomoreawareness.org
Co-founders: Janet Morana and Georgette Forney
A campaign whereby Christians make the public aware of
the devastation abortion brings to women and men. The
campaign **seeks to expose and heal the secrecy and
silence surrounding the emotional and physical pain
of abortion.** Silent No More reaches out to people hurt by
abortion, encouraging them to attend abortion after-care
programs. Invite those who are ready to break the silence
to join them. There are 2,943 testimonies posted on their
campaign website with 618 that are shared via video. **248
women are listed whose deaths are documented as being
caused by abortion.**

Suicide Prevention Lifeline: 800 273-8255
https://suicidepreventionlifeline.org/

The Abortion Survivors Network:
https://theabortionsurvivors.com/
Stories from babies who survived abortion.

UNPLANNED:
https://www.unplannedfilm.com/contact-us
The life story of Abby Johnson, former Planned Parenthood
executive. Learn why she became disillusioned with Planned
Parenthood and is wonderfully pro-life. The first month after
this film was released, 500 current abortion facility employees
called their helpline to discuss resigning their jobs. Abby
Johnson also has a sister organization for **abortion workers
who want to leave the industry:**
And Then There Were None
www.abortionworker.com
888-570-1588

Wendy's Wonderful Kids®:
https://www.davethomasfoundation.org/
The Foundation works closely with child welfare advocates
and policymakers, *provides free resources about foster care
adoption and raises awareness through social media campaigns,
public service announcements and events.* (If you want to adopt a
foster child, contact them to see if they might help you.)

Media outlets typically describe the numbers of late-term abortions as "very rare". They cite the fact that they only account for 1.3 percent of all abortions. There are more than 12,000 reported abortions annually after 20 weeks of pregnancy. (https://www.nejm.org/doi/full/10.1056/NEJMsri804754) Let's consider other ways children die annually: 4,000 from car crashes, 3,000 from gun violence, 2,000 from childhood cancers. Each of these tragic numbers represents only a fraction of the deaths from late term abortions. One of the most horrendous abortionists had a clinic in Pennsylvania, a state which outlawed abortion if the baby was over 24 weeks old, the age they deemed the child could live. You can enter Kermit Gosnell in your search engine. His staff admitted that 40% of his abortions were done on babies who were more than 24 weeks old. He was convicted of murder and sentenced to life in prison plus 30 years.

HOW TO STOP PERSONS WISHING TO VOTE FROM HOME FROM GETTING DUPLICATE BALLOTS

The key is instead of indiscriminate mailing out of ballots, voters will only get a ballot if they mail in a request for one. Voters will send in a SASE (Self-Addressed-Stamped-Envelope) Voters will also include their birthday, address on file with their precinct, printed name and signature. If their address has changed, they will update it.

When the poll worker gets the envelope, they will check the postmark to make certain it was mailed in on time. They will video each step. They will pull the signature on file up on their computer and compare it to the signature mailed in. If it matches, they will mail the voter their ballot and a postpaid return envelope which states the postage is only paid if used by X date. If the ballot request is denied an explanation will be sent. This procedure will be saved in the computer and made available to those auditing the procedure. Persons violating these guidelines will be charged with a felony, fined $1,000 per incident, be prohibited from voting for five years and be identified on the internet. The chemicals in the ink and colors used to print ballots may be slightly altered by precinct so counterfeits can be identified and disqualified. Persons possessing and/or submitting more than one ballot will be given the same penalties and fined $1,000 per ballot. Groups of consecutive ballots cast for the same candidate will not exceed 20 ballots unless the authorities can prove it is mathematically possible for there to be huge numbers of ballots all being consecutively cast for the same candidate.

BONUS APPENDIX WHICH SHOWS YOU THE TRUE CHARACTER OF GOD – WHEN YOU NEED A GOOD SAMARITAN (Luke 10)

Jesus got along great with the common people. But some of the Jewish religious leaders were jealous of his success. They tried again and again to catch him saying something which was inconsistent with their Scriptures. Therefore we read about Jesus being put to the test by a religious leader who asks, *"Teacher what must I do to inherit eternal life?"*

This parable speaks to the question about how we are given eternal life.

And Jesus said to him, *"What is written in the laws?"* (Remember, our Jewish friends frequently answer a question with a question. Jesus asked 287 questions in the four gospels. One Gentile asked his Jewish buddy, "Why do you insist on answering my questions to you with a question?" His friend shrugged his shoulders and said, "Why not?" I have heard that in all but two conversations recorded in Scriptures, Jesus answers a question with a question.)

And He answered and said, *"You shall love the Lord your God with all your heart, and with all your strength, and with all your mind, and your neighbor as yourself"* (Deuteronomy 6:5).

And Jesus said, *"You have answered correctly. Do this and you shall live."*

But wishing to justify himself, he asked Jesus, *"And who is my neighbor?"*

The religious lawyer mistakenly thought one has to "do" something to "inherit" eternal life, to go to heaven. Jesus knew that no one does anything to receive an inheritance. An inheritance is a gift. *"For by grace you have been saved through faith. It is a gift of God, not a result of works, lest any man should boast"* (Ephesians 2:8). *Grace means to get something we don't deserve.* We don't deserve salvation. *Mercy means not to get something we do deserve.* We do deserve eternal punishment. If you are uninsured and crash your car into the back of my car and I don't sue you to make you pay for my vehicle and bodily injury damages, I would be treating you with mercy. **If on the other hand, because your car was totaled in the accident you caused, if I bought you the gift of a new car, that would be grace.** (See also Psalm 100:5) *"Grace and truth came by Jesus Christ"* (John 1:17).

The use of parables was prophesied. (Psalms 78:2; Matthew 13:34).

Jesus used parables. **A parable is an earthly story with a heavenly meaning.** So, Jesus either related or devised a situation where a person who was totally helpless still gets saved from his problem: Jesus replied, *"A certain man was going down from Jerusalem to Jericho.* (Jericho is the lowest city in the world. It is 833 feet below sea level. The distance from Jerusalem to Jericho is 24 miles. Jerusalem is 1,800 feet higher than Jericho.) *And he fell among robbers, and they stripped him and beat him, and went off leaving him half dead."*

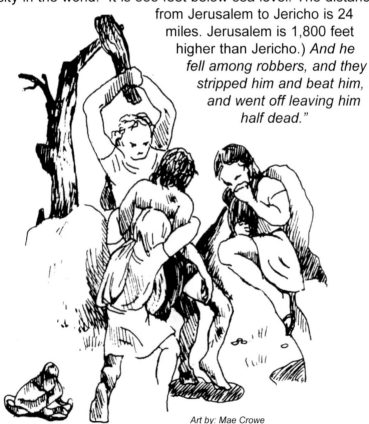

Art by: Mae Crowe

The victim had no clothes, no valuables with which to buy help, and was beaten within an inch of his life. He could not solve his own problem and needed help. And, he knew it.

Because he was Jewish, the victim no doubt prayed to God. He might even have imagined that the ideal person to help him would be a full-time religious worker rather than a lay person. You might have heard this joke, "A religious worker gets paid to do good. A lay person is good for nothing". So, certainly this victim was relieved at what he saw coming. We read: *"And by chance a certain priest was going down that road, and when he saw him, passed by on the other side. And likewise a levite also, when he came to the place and saw him, passed by on the other side."* He might even have recognized these two and they might have known him.

The priest and levite lived off tithes and offerings of men like the beaten up Jewish merchant. But, this helpless man who no doubt contributed to the livelihood of these supposedly God fearing men, found out his religion didn't help him. Does your religion help you with the biggest problems of your life? If it doesn't, you might be wise to consider a creative alternative. **Religion is an organization. Christianity is a relationship.**

These religious men did not obey their own laws, *"Love your neighbor as yourself"* (Leviticus 19:10). They didn't practice what they preached. To try and justify their own merciless behavior, these men might have assumed that had they stopped to help the dying merchant and had he died on them, they would not have been able to work in the temple until after some days of cleansing themselves, because they would have become unclean by touching a dead body. Yet, none of us can fail to see it is more important to save a life than to perform in a synagogue, temple, church or mosque. Terrorists today sometimes attack those who come to help rescue victims of terrorism. The priest and levite knew that if they stopped, they may also be ambushed by the same thieves.

When you need a Good Samaritan

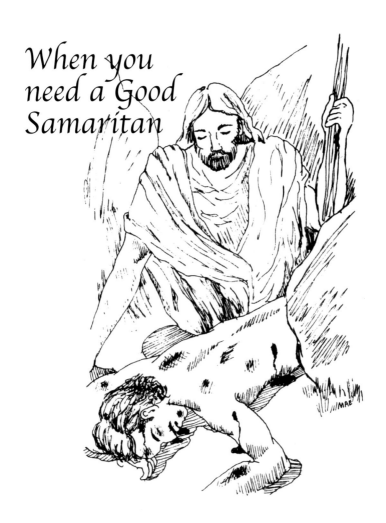

"But a certain Samaritan, who was on a journey, came upon him and when he saw him, he felt compassion and came to him, and bandaged up his wounds, pouring oil and wine on them, and he put him on his own beast, and brought him to an inn, and took care of him."

Samaritans were part Jew and part Gentile. Jews hated and looked down on them so much that when they went from Galilee (North Israel) to Judea (South Israel), they frequently walked around Samaria (Central Israel). So, the Jewish merchant had no expectation of help from the approaching Samaritan. But, when the Samaritan saw the dying merchant, *"He felt compassion and came to him."*

Sympathy is to feel for. Empathy is to feel with. Compassion is to act on one's feelings. The two religious men possibly had perfect feelings towards the dying victim, but nothing they felt helped him.

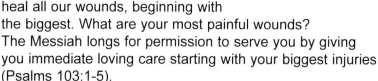

When Jesus the Great Physician looks at us, the first thing He notices are our wounds. My favorite current TV drama is "The Good Doctor." Doctors are not turned off by injuries. In fact, the worse an injury is, the more interesting, the more intriguing it is to a medical doctor. Jesus is the Great and Complete Physician. Jesus wants to heal all our wounds, beginning with the biggest. What are your most painful wounds? The Messiah longs for permission to serve you by giving you immediate loving care starting with your biggest injuries (Psalms 103:1-5).

So also, THE GOOD SAMARITAN came to him and poured wine on the wounds, because it has alcohol, an antiseptic to prevent infection. The Good Samaritan also poured on oil because it promotes healing. Then he bound the wounds, to protect them from further injury. *"They that are whole don't need a physician, but they that are sick do"* (Luke 5:31 see also Luke 4:23).

The reason you are holding this book right now is because THE GOOD SAMARITAN has come to you. If you have been wounded, know that he is also longing to treat your wounds. Will you let him dress your visible and invisible wounds? He also longs to take His big handkerchief out of His back pocket and *"wipe away all tears from our eyes"* (Revelation 21:4).

The father of one of my high school classmates had a road construction business. He nearly lost it and much more, because he was an alcoholic. Once this man came to my father and said, "I am sorry I am at the end of my rope." My father smiled and explained, "You need not apologize, that is where Jesus wants you to be." Moments later, this man believed in the Messiah. Some time afterwards, his health and business were also restored.

If the creation that we know about so far were the size of the Pacific Ocean, earth would be the size of the head of a common pin. James 4:16 says, *"You are just a vapor that appears for a little while and then vanishes away."* So, you and I are a mist on the head of a pin in the middle of a Pacific Ocean sized creation. How could we ever find the eternal God, especially when we are like the nearly murdered merchant, naked, broke and half dead?

Matthew 18:11 reveals Jesus' mission. *"For the Son of Man has come to save that which was lost."* Jesus explains that His love is like that of a Good Shepherd, who leaves his flock of ninety-nine sheep and searches until he finds one lost lamb (Matthew 18:12ff). (Note: The Messiah has a special concern for the young).

Some people say, "I can't believe in the Messiah. I would fall into sin." Can you imagine the Good Samaritan not holding the man up when he clothed, traded places with him and put him on his own beast? The inn is the synagogue or church, the fellowship of believers. The man was taken to the inn, where he recovered. Because the merchant was penniless, we read, *"And on the next day the Good Samaritan took out two day's wages (2 denari) and gave them to the innkeeper and said, "Take care of him: and whatever more you spend, when I return, I will repay you."* The denarius was the most common Roman coin used in Jesus Christ's day. It represented an average of one day's wages.

Ephesians 1:8 reads, "In Jesus we have redemption through His blood, the forgiveness of our trespasses, according to the riches of His grace which He lavished upon us." Jesus pays for our sins with His blood (see also Isaiah 53:6). Romans 6:23 explains that we need a death to pay for our sins. *"For the wages of sin is death, but the free gift of God is eternal life in Christ Jesus our Lord."*

Finally, the Good Samaritan says He will return to pay the injured man's total debt. In the same way Jesus has paid our total sin debt. Jesus is coming back, when we don't expect it, *"like a thief in the night"* (I Thessalonians 5:2). Let's conclude the parable. And Jesus asked him, *"Which of these three men, the priest, the levite or the Good Samaritan prove to be a neighbor to the man who was attacked by robbers?"* The man who questioned Jesus answered, *"I suppose the one who showed mercy to the one who was attacked."* Jesus said to him, *"Go and do likewise"* (As recorded in Luke 10:30-37). By protecting the unborn and their mothers, we are fulfilling the Lord's command to *"go and do likewise."*

Are you ready for life? For death? For the Messiah's soon return? To be ready, you need to believe in the Messiah. Becoming a believer is such a radical event, Jesus calls it being *"born again"* (John 3). A Christian is a repentant and forgiven sinner with Christ in his or her heart. Suppose you were about to jump off a diving board head first into an empty pool. If you were to repent of doing this foolish act, you would stop moving toward the end of the diving board, turn around and get off the board. The Bible says, *"Thou shalt not kill"* (Exodus 20:16). If you were in the business of killing unborn children what actions could you take to repent? You would walk away from that career and become pro-life in thought word and deed. Jesus warned, *"Except you repent (stop sinning), you will all likewise perish"* (Luke 13:3). Repentant people turn from evil to walk in light, not darkness (1 John 1).

MY FAVORITE ILLUSTRATION IN THIS BOOK
A young pastor began serving at a church which had a woman with a unique reputation. She claimed she could hear from God. The pastor asked his bishop how to deal with this person. The bishop personally came to test her claims. He asked, "The night I graduated from college I unfortunately committed a sin. Please next time God talks with you, ask him what that sin was." The woman agreed. Not long afterwards

the bishop returned to the parish and asked the woman to identify that sin. The woman smiled and reported, "God said He didn't remember your sin."

"I am He who blots out your transgressions, for My own sake, and remembers your sins no more" (Isaiah 43:25). *"For I will forgive their wickedness and will remember their sins no more"* (Hebrews 8:12).

1 John 1:9 explains how to get forgiveness, *"If we confess our sins, He is faithful and just to forgive us our sins and to cleanse us from all unrighteousness."* Sins which are not confessed and forsaken damn us to an eternal hell (Luke 17:26).

*"Then I acknowledged my sin to you and did not cover up my iniquity. **I said, 'I will confess my transgressions to the** Lord.' And you forgave the guilt of my sin"* (Psalm 32:5).

To welcome the Messiah into your life, follow Revelation 3:20 (Messiah speaking). *"Behold I stand at the door and knock, if any man hear My voice and open the door, I will come in to him and sup with him and he with Me."* In the Jewish culture, the most intimate thing you could do with someone would be to have them over for dinner. **That's another reason why the Jewish leaders were so torqued with Jesus. He not only was a friend to tax collectors and sinners, He dined with them!** (For further details see Matthew 9:10). You may have seen the famous painting of the Messiah standing outside the door to a person's heart knocking. The artist was criticized for omitting the handle on the outside of the door. The artist smiled and explained, "The latch is on the inside." The Messiah is a gentleman. He will not force Himself on any person. *"Love does not insist on its own way"* (1 Corinthians 13). *"God is love"* (John 4:7-21).

SOME OF YOU MY DEAR FRIENDS HAVE MISUSED YOUR HANDS – BE ENCOURAGED

"All those who the Father gives Me will come to Me. Him who comes to Me I will in no way cast out" (John 6:37). He is especially jealous to win the love of those who want to repent and need to be forgiven many sins. *"Therefore I tell you, her sins, which are many, are forgiven—for she loved much. But he who is forgiven little, loves little"* (Luke 7:47). *"Draw near to God and He will draw near to you. **Cleanse your hands, you sinners; and purify your hearts, you double-minded"** (James 4:8).* Luke 15 tells how when the prodigal son finally *"came to himself and returned home, while he was yet a great way off, his father saw him, and had compassion and ran to him, and fell on his neck and kissed him,"* etc. (The Old Testament prescribed severe penalties when children disobeyed or gave dishonor to their parents. The possibility exists that the neighbors of the father of the Prodigal Son had their eye out for him. And when they caught him trying to return home, they might have planned on catching and stoning him to death. Maybe this was why the father was looking for his son and ran to him. He wanted to keep him from being killed by the citizens of their community. The father also gave him the best robe, a ring and killed the fatted calf throwing him a fabulous welcome home party. This parable celebrates the power of forgiveness. The father in the story represents our Heavenly Father. Let us celebrate the welcome God gives repentant sinners. May we all accept the gifts which come to those who stop sinning and ask for forgiveness.)

God is looking for, and is eager to run to receive you. Please give Him the chance. Then you can know you have eternal life. *"Therefore go and make disciples of all nations, baptizing them in the name of the Father and of the Son and of the Holy Spirit, and teaching them to obey everything I have commanded you. And surely I am with you always, to the very end of the age"* (Matthew 28:19-20). *"Anyone who believes and is baptized will be saved. But anyone who refuses to believe will be condemned"* (Mark 16:16). (See also 1 John 5:12.)

Eternal life starts the moment you believe in the Messiah. *"What are the game plans of Satan (also called "the thief") and Jesus? "The thief comes only to steal, kill and destroy. I came that they may have life and have it more abundantly"* (John 10:10). All those involved in the lucrative abortion industry work to fulfill Satan's game plan. They will also receive Satan's reward for their choices. On judgment day Jesus will tell the ungodly, *"Depart from Me you who are accused, into the eternal fire prepared for the devil and his angels"* (Matthew 25:41). The list of things the accursed did includes this, ***"I was sick and you did not look after Me...whatever you did not do for one of the least of these, you did not do for Me. Then they will go away to eternal punishment, but the righteous to eternal life"*** (Matthew 25:45, 46). You can control if you follow Christ or Satan, but you cannot control the consequences of your choice.

Women in an unplanned pregnancy are included in the category of *"those who are sick."* Let us reach out in tenderness and love to help them. Many of the pro-life resources in this book are also faith based. Reach out to them. Please refer to the extensive list of organizations in the resource section. I believe no matter what your background is, you will be able to find a group with whom you can share and be helped.

Unborn children and their natural and adopted parents thank you that you agreed to CHOOSE LIFE! *"First seek the counsel of the Lord"* (1 Kings 22:5).

IS NAPRO TECHNOLOGY MORE EFFECTIVE IN OVERCOMING INFERTILITY THAN IVF?

Dr. Anne Nolte practices at the Giana Center For Women's Health and Fertility in Manhattan, New York City. She explained that 95 percent of the couples who come to her with difficulty conceiving or who are suffering recurrent miscarriages have no diagnosis when they arrive. Using NaPro Technology® (Natural Procreative Technology is a proven women's health science that monitors and maintains a woman's reproductive and gynecological health.) The majority of them have their problem diagnosed and treated and are able to conceive and carry to term. "Our success rate is as good as or better than IVF (in vitro fertilization). And we have very low rates of multiple births and...of birth defects." (Source: RECALL ABORTIONS by Janet Morana, p.61ff.)

During IVF, the eggs are fertilized in a petri dish. Multiple fertilized eggs are then implanted in the mother in the hope that at least one healthy one will survive. As the pregnancy progresses, excess fertilized eggs are frequently unfortunately destroyed. It is too bad that during this procedure the creation of a wanted child comes at the expense of creating and ending the life of one or more unwanted children. To find a medical consultant like Dr. Nolte, go to www.fertilitycare.org.

EPILOGUE

Life is not a DVD to be popped into a machine and played again at will. **Life is a one time shot and will not be repeated.** God help us make the most of it. Life is not a rehearsal. *"For he says, 'In a favorable time I listened to you, and in a day of salvation I have helped you.' Behold, now is the favorable time; behold, now is the day of salvation"* (2 Corinthians 6:2). *"This is the day the Lord has made; let us rejoice and be glad in it"* (Psalm 118:24).

While reading this book, one of my close friends commented that there are so many negative aspects to abortion she felt nearly overwhelmed. *To her the most significant reason to be pro-life is that it enables us to celebrate the miracle of birth.* Let's put things in perspective. Imagine the joys of life, love and being a family! So my friends, let's pass arm in arm through the door marked life.

Thank you for reading my poems and allowing me to share my research and philosophy.

I hope to secure funds so this book can be freely given away to those entering crisis pregnancy facilities. May my words cause any of you my dear readers who are deciding whether or not to have an abortion, to CHOOSE LIFE. Study the resource section and reach out for help.

If you have a loved one or good friend experiencing a crisis pregnancy, by all means consider being the person who says, "I will stand by you!" in their time of need. And share this book. Information about how to read it on line will soon be available (p.2).

And to you our friends who have been working in the abortion industry, we hope and pray you join us. Enough babies have died. It is time for life and for you to use your God given skill to support rather than to end life.

WHO COMMANDS WE CHOOSE LIFE?

When my son was four and he and I were renting from my parents, mom was watching through the kitchen window and listening to my son and his best friend David play in the back yard. David suggested they do something which was wrong. My son refused. David kept bugging him to do it. Finally, my son put his hands on his hips and said, "David, don't you want to be on the winning side?" My son explained that when everything was said and done, God will judge us and we need to do the right thing. This argument persuaded David to stop encouraging my son to do the questionable activity. For you my dear readers, I give you the same question, "Don't you want to be on the winning side?" We reap what we sow.

Moses laid it out clearly for the Jewish nation, *"This day I call heaven and earth to witness against you, that I have set before you life and death, blessing and curses. Now **choose life, so that you and your children may live** and that you may love the Lord your God, listen to His voice, and hold fast to Him. For the Lord is your life, and He will give you many years in the land He swore to give your fathers, Abraham, Isaac and Jacob"* (Deuteronomy 30:19-20). *"Children are a gift from the Lord; they are a reward from Him. Children born to a young man are like arrows in a warrior's hands. How joyful is the man whose quiver is full of them! He will not be put to shame when he confronts his accusers at the city gates"* (Psalm 127:3-5). (The well lived life of your family will silence the criticisms of your accusers.)

The fundamental medical precept of Hypocrites is *"primum non nocere"* which is Latin for "First do no harm." Now I have reported my observations about the honesty of abortionists when they claim they provide a safe abortion. You may decide if they can be trusted and are telling the truth.

I switched my major when I was at Augsburg from English to pre-med and ended up earning degrees in speech and music. The next question was, *"What should I do for a career?"* I had a strong impression that I should send an unsolicited manuscript to the largest circulating religious periodical in the world. Billy

Graham's Minneapolis based DECISION MAGAZINE had twice the circulation of the next largest magazine. I sensed that if the editor encouraged me to be a Christian writer that would be the way I should go. And vice versa. So I wrote one paragraph of commentary on each of two Scriptures and sent it in to DECISION. Two days later I had a note in my PO Box 557 at Augsburg College to call Sherwood Wirt, Editor. He said, "Dale, I enjoyed your submission. Would you care to drop by tomorrow at 11:00 so we could talk?" I told him "I think I can work that in." He added, "If you have any other writing samples, please bring them along." He graciously gave me an hour of his time, copied a half inch stack of my writing samples and said in essence "Dale, be a writer." It turns out he knew my mom because they both belonged to the Minnesota Christian Writers Guild where he was president. He gave me a scholarship for the DECISION MAGAZINE CHRISTIAN WRITERS INSTITUTE the next summer. Then he pressed the intercom and invited the associate editor, Lois Weigand to come in. She bought me lunch, took a personal interest in me, and over a two hour period said in essence, "Dale be a writer!"

When I stepped outside after the meal I looked to heaven and said, **"In three days I had three hours with the top two people in the number one best selling Christian magazine in the world saying I should be a writer. Maybe You're trying to tell me something?"**

One of the poems I gave Dr. Wirt that day is in this book, "She Must Be Yours." God answered this prayer for a wife 15 months later after my first year of grad school. I hit the jackpot and was given Miss Felton, to be my amazing brilliant beautiful wife. She had nine months left to finish her degree in Anesthesiology.

The Lord has plans for every child in the womb. The plans were in place before they were even conceived. Is that great or what? **Aren't you dying to know how your unborn child will turn out?** Each of us has a God planned destiny. For sure if you are expecting, God has plans for your child. I am writing this during 2021. Let's seek God's guidance in all decisions regarding our present, unborn and future family. *"For I know the plans I have for you, declares the LORD, plans to prosper you and not to harm you, to give you a future and a hope"* (Jeremiah 29:11).

GEMS FROM JACK HAYFORD

In his book I'LL HOLD YOU IN HEAVEN, Jack Hayford writes, *"The way He overcame sin was by surrendering himself to love — to stand forgiving before sin until His love overcame it."* (p.106)

"Inherent in every child is not only the promise of God's purpose but the provision of God's power to accomplish that purpose." (p.52)

"Depersonalizing feelings are often accentuated when people discover they are illegitimate offspring or the product of an extramarital affair. Individuals question their worth, despair over their destiny and often succumb to feelings of pointlessness - especially in a society that argues for chance as the explanation of man's existence rather than God's purpose." (p.54)

How can we instill a feeling of self worth when a parent tells his child, "You were not planned." Or tells the youngest child, "I wish we would have had fewer children." The key is to get the child to understand that **even before he or she was conceived, God had already planned out important things that they would be doing with their life. Therefore God's plan for them takes precedence over any** negative feelings their parents might have towards them. As we discover and follow God's plan for our life, we come to realize the tremendous value each of us has.

The subtitle of Hayford's book is, "Healing and hope for the parent who has lost a child through miscarriage, stillbirth, abortion or early infant death." He asks, "What happens to my baby after he or she died? Will I ever see my baby again - and will I recognize him? What happens if I've had an abortion? Does God have a reason for letting my child die? How can I help a friend who is in grief?"

250,000 of this remarkable book are in print. I plan on further studying and learning from this book. I just got it recently. But I wanted to let you know it exists. Of one thing Hayford is certain, if you lost a child in these four categories **your child is in heaven** and if you have given your life to and trust in Jesus, **you will reunite with, recognize and be able to interact with your infant**. It has comforted grieving parents and will encourage you.

A certain mother was an evolutionist and taught her children that man was descended from monkeys. The father was a creationist and believed God created us. The children came to the father and asked, "So, Dad, which view is right?" The father said. "Both of us. Your mother's side of the family came from monkeys. And my side came from God." Oh, the beauty of compromise!

Have you heard the latest definition of an evolutionist? "Someone who can trace his family tree all the way back to the tree, when they were swinging monkeys."

John describes the future God has prepared for us in heaven by saying, *"Now the dwelling of God is with men. He will live with them. They will be His people. And God Himself will be with them and be their God. He will wipe every tear from their eyes. There will be no more death or mourning or crying, or pain. For the old order of things has passed away. He who is seated on the throne said, 'I am making everything new'"* (Revelation 21:3-6). (See also Isaiah 35. Meditate on the whole chapter and be encouraged.)

I distinctly remember a thought which came to me when I was in choir rehearsal when I was 18 and we were singing the anthem, *"Surely He has born our griefs and carried our sorrow"* (Isaiah 53;6). I raised my hand and Ruth Nelson the director called on me. I said, "If the Lord has done this, what do we have left?" The bottom line my dear reader is this, "We don't want to miss out on the amazing plans God has for us and our children."

MAKE LOVE YOUR CHOICE

With what has God entrusted you
    my special pregnant friend?
Your life has limitless potential.
You can send

    this life into the future...as
    an archer bends her bow.
The arrow from your quiver can
    sail true. Or you can go

    into a place where childrens' lives
    are deemed worthless. They're trash.
Abortionists stick out their palms,
    ask for your hard earned cash.

The irresponsible trend we all have
    bids you to walk away.
To throw your bow and arrow down
    until a better day.

Look in the mirror. You child exists
    and looks to you with love.
Will you discard this precious gift
    given from the Lord above?

The world waits for your child. Her worth
    is priceless. Soon her birth
    will affirm you have a mother's heart
Check out your gorgeous girth.

Your little one reaches out with trust
    expectantly. Don't bail.
Accept the challenge. Be brave and strong.
Be giving. Sweet. Don't fail.

Your lips are made to kiss your child.
Your arms are made for hugs.
Your child will be inquisitive,
    love mud puddles and bugs.

The mysteries of things that you can share Mom
      is so grand.
All that you need to do is reach out now
      and take her by the hand.

She'll be a cutie. Give you joy,
      and you will be fulfilled.
The Lord has so much waiting for you.
Your cup will not be spilled.

Psalm 23 explains instead your cup
      will overflow. Step up and meet the test.
His goodness and His mercy wait.
He'll give you what is best.

God offers love also to those who
      are abortionists.
They misinterpret freedom's truths.
They are contortionists.

Reach out to those who wish to end
      the lives of the unborn.
The time has come for them to change.
And for their sins to mourn.

When they choose life and change their ways
      your arrow will be sent.
And God will welcome them with love,
      when they bow and repent.

Each day has options, pick yours well.
Be wise and use your voice.
Bring as many as you can to life.
Always make love your choice!

"So abide faith, hope and love, these three, but the greatest of
these is love" (I Corinthians 13:13).

THAT UNBORN MAY LIVE!

What goal do I have for this book of poems?
THAT UNBORN MAY LIVE! Hear deep breaths and moans.
Push cherished life through the birth canal.
Let's vote life! Little One we all tell you,
W E L C O M E!!

IF SOMEONE YOU DEEPLY CARE ABOUT HAS AN UNEXPECTED PREGNANCY

Don't ask, "So what will you do now?" Why? Because that implies they might consider having an abortion.

The best of many responses I have heard follows. "Well, you have an 'unexpected blessing.' Is there anything I might do to help you as you plan for the wellbeing of your child?"

Now remember the most important statistic in this book. Over half the women who chose to have an abortion reported, "If someone, anyone, the father, a friend, or family member would have told me, I will stand by you as you carry your child, I would not have had the abortion." Armed with this statistic, we who love life can unite and reduce the number of abortions in our beloved America by over half. Can you who love life think of a more important task? Why not tell the Lord, "If you want me to stand by a woman in an unexpected pregnancy, open the door so I can meet this woman and I will give my word that I will make a deliberate effort to stand by her."

You might even contact a counseling service near you and explain that, "Even if I don't know the woman, if you have one who needs someone to stand by her, you may put me in touch with her and I will stand by her." Approximately one of every three women over 45 in America have had an abortion. I am thinking that for a woman who has had one and genuinely regrets doing so, to befriend and stand by a woman who births her unborn child might also help her heal from her mistake. You will notice in the resource section there are organizations which train caring folks how to support a woman in a crisis pregnancy. Study the resource section and take intentional steps to help women and couples CHOOSE LIFE.

GIVING ABORTIONISTS THE LAST WORD

The following quotes were taken from the best book I ever read on the subject, Janet Morana's publication called RECALL ABORTION, Chapter two.

Phyllis from Ohio wrote of her abortion, I never saw the abortion doctor until just before the procedure. I was reluctant to let him go in with the instruments. **He said, jokingly, "Just spread your legs like a cheerleader."** I did not laugh. The nurse who promised to hold my hand was very warm and kind until they turned on the suction. Then her hand went limp, like she did not want to touch me. I pray for her sometimes. I cried when it was done, but I was so out of touch from blocking my feelings about it, that I really don't know what I was crying about. I don't remember my pain. I do remember the blank faces of all the women in the recovery room. They looked so deflated.

Jodi of Illinois had an abortion at fourteen and another at sixteen. During the second one she said, "I was crying the whole time. So much was running through my mind and I wanted to leave so badly, but I didn't. As I was lying on the table, I felt so humiliated. **The doctor looked at me and said to the nurse, 'Oh, we'll see this one here again.'** I looked at him and said, 'You will never see me again.' He laughed and replied, 'Yeah, right. That's what they all say.' I felt so alone and afraid."

Kim in Mississippi was also mistreated at the abortion clinic. **"After taking a sedative and being strapped down to the exam table I said, 'I can't do this. Let me up.' After that I was forcefully held down by two people** and given another sedative, this time an injection into my hand. I put my legs together and heard the doctor tell the assistant to do something about that. They held my legs apart and I begged

233

and called for my boyfriend. Today, I know that he never heard my screams. The doctor started the procedure and I felt pain and could hear the suction noise. I felt sick and could feel the hot tears flowing down my face. I just wanted to die."

In Kentucky, Vicki fared no better. "At the abortion clinic, we were given no counseling. They gave us a standard medical form to fill out and that was it. No one discussed with us we had other options or parenting. They just asked about our money. **When the procedure began I asked the doctor to stop and he said to me, 'You should have thought of that before you got yourself knocked up.'** I have never been so poorly treated in my entire life."

Nancy Zevgolis is a nurse who exercised her rights of conscience to avoid taking part in an abortion. She helped prepare the operating room. A young Orthodox Jewish couple, told their baby's heart problems would prove fatal, made the decision to abort after eight-and-a-half months. She writes, "You could see it was hard on them and I remember thinking, 'Just have the baby and see what happens, you never know.'"

Although she said she would not scrub for the procedure, when her replacement didn't arrive and the patient was under anesthesia, she said, "I couldn't leave. I let it go too far." Years later she said the image is seared into her memory. **The doctor, his foot on the bottom of the operating room table to get better leverage tearing a full-term baby apart piece by piece with his forceps.** It comes back to haunt me. The bloody abortion took about twenty minutes. When it was over both she and the other nurse in the room were crying. The parents had to have the baby's parts for a Jewish burial, and Ms. Zevgolis found herself guarding the remains and hand carrying them up to pathology. She got dressed and left after that, never returning to that hospital again. But the memories will never leave her. Almost a decade later she still struggles to comprehend the brutality she witnessed. As a devout Catholic she went to confession. But adds, "Even now I still don't feel clean because I took part in it. It just really bothers me in my heart and soul."

SUPERB COUNSELOR'S TECHNIQUE – THE ABORTIONIST'S PSALM

A tremendously successful counselor would start his sessions by listening to the person's problems. Then he would ask, "Please give me a little time." He would close his eyes and silently pray to the Lord to guide him. Then he would open his bible to a place where a person was facing a similar temptation or challenge. Fast forward to the specific thing which an abortionist does. What method do abortionists use to extract a child from the womb? As the child grows, his or her size presents a challenge for the surgeon. I recently discovered a Psalm which explains the abortionist's dilemma. The key passage is Psalms 7:1-2, *"O Lord my God, I take refuge in You. Save and deliver me from all who pursue me.* OR **THEY WILL TEAR ME LIKE A LION, AND RIP ME TO PIECES WITH NO ONE TO RESCUE ME...**" (Note: one of my goals in writing this book is to motivate brave caring people to "rescue" children living in their mother's womb. In the opening paragraphs of this book I promised to identify the weaknesses of our opponents.) *"HE WHO IS PREGNANT WITH EVIL AND CONCEIVES TROUBLE GIVES BIRTH TO DISILLUSIONMENT. HE WHO DIGS A HOLE AND SCOOPS IT OUT FALLS INTO THE PIT HE HAS MADE. THE TROUBLE HE CAUSES RECOILS ON HIMSELF. HIS VIOLENCE COMES DOWN ON HIS OWN HEAD"* (Psalms 7:14-16). Abortionists are wrong when they presume they can continue to kill the unborn. If a woman is pregnant, unless someone ends her pregnancy or she has a miscarriage, she will give birth. Abortionists are similarly pregnant. 100% of them will learn they are wrong. Then they have a choice to stop doing wrong, repent and ask God's mercy, or to face God's eternal wrath. May we who love life not stop until we succeed in helping our friends in the abortion industry admit they were disillusioned and to CHOOSE LIFE!

WHY PURSUE THE YES LIFE?

To say yes to the world God invites us to enter is obedience, emptying of self, surrendering control, to live in the palm of

Christ's nail scarred hand forever. To know God's presence every moment is a privilege and honor few pay the full price to experience. To say yes seems simple to me but to others it is full of peril and reluctance. Yes can be painful - sharp corners poking me in my emotions, upsetting my equilibrium, unbalancing thoughts, creating wants. Self arises to complain about being poked by the sharp edges of yes. I would not desire a before yes life. THE INCREDIBLE RIDE ON THE CREST OF GOD'S POWER FLOWING THROUGH ME IS HEAVEN NOW! (Elizabeth Everitt)

A parting encouraging promise for those of you my friends who miss your unborn child. "Absence diminishes weak passions and increases great ones, as the wind blows out candles and fans fires." Francois de La Rouchefoucauld, 1665

A PRESCHOOLER ASKS HER MOM THE ULTIMATE QUESTION

The following illustration was shared by Pastor Peter Franz on September 13, 2020. A mother mentioned to her bright inquisitive daughter that one of their elderly family members had died. Her daughter asked, "Mommy did she go to heaven?" Her mom was happy to explain that, "Yes, she loved and trusted in Jesus. She is safely in heaven now." Then one by one the little girl mentioned the names of other family members and asked, "Are they going to heaven?" The mother gave her best estimate of their relationship with Jesus.

The little girl thanked her mom. Then she added, "I am going to heaven when I die. I know. I talked to Jesus on the phone."

Her mom asked, "How did you know Jesus' phone number?" Her daughter's face radiated joy and she explained, "Mommy, Jesus called me!"

Prayer is talking with God. IS YOUR PHONE RINGING? Hebrews 2:3 asks, *"How shall we escape if we ignore such a great salvation?"*

"In fact, God is patient, because He wants everyone to turn from sin and no one to be lost… and would have no man to perish, but would all men to come to repentance…" (2 Peter 3:9).

God promises, *"Whoever comes to Me I will in no way cast out"* (John 6:37).

"If we endure, we shall also reign with Him. If we deny Him He will also deny us. If we are faithless, He remains faithful, for He cannot deny Himself" (II Timothy 2:12, 13).

A certain atheistic grandfather was in a hospice with only a short time left to live. Most of his family members loved Jesus. When they would visit, many would encourage him to trust Jesus to forgive his sins, cleanse him and make his peace with God. Frankly he was sick and tired of being nagged about his relationship with the Lord. So he asked the nurses for a large sheet of paper and magic marker and wrote a big sign and taped it to his wall. The sign said, GOD IS NOWHERE. Fortunately this grandfather had a seven year old granddaughter who loved him unconditionally and did not bug him about his relationship with God. He reveled in the acceptance of little Cindy. (By the way Cindy means literally, moon or moon goddess. The spiritual meaning is "Reflector of God's light.") When Cindy had given her grandfather a big happy to see you hug and smooch, she took a full minute to study the sign. A smile appeared on her face and she excitedly said, "Grandpa, I am so happy! You also believe in Jesus?" He laughed and asked, "Why do you think I do?" She pointed to and sounded out the sign phonetically, "God is now here!"

This unconditional love of his favorite granddaughter broke through the wall of his unbelief...and in that moment HE PICKED UP THE PHONE and Jesus welcomed him into the family of God. We Christians are not always smooth in our approach to sharing our faith. I recall Bill Bright saying, **"If, after I share the gospel with you, you still don't believe it, it is because I have failed to present it clearly enough."** I hope and pray my sharing my faith...and the testimony of the two granddaughters in these concluding illustrations have melted your heart. My friends, even if you had an honorable job or were making mega bucks in the abortion industry...if you gained the whole world, when you die it would profit you nothing.

When I was young, I noticed my grandmother studying her Bible with great intensity. I asked, "Why are you spending so much time reading the bible? She explained, "I am cramming for my finals." When I was a full time student, when I was preparing for a test, I would try to anticipate the questions the teacher would ask. In Hebrews 9:27 it says, *"It is given to man once to die and then comes the judgment."* My father used to say, "When we stand before almighty God, we will not be judged by what we think the Bible says or what others have told us it says. They could be wrong. We will be judged by what it actually says. So we best know what it says." I believe God will ask me, **"Dale, have you sinned?"** I will have to say, "Yes, Romans 3:23 explains, *all have sinned and fallen short of the glory of God."* Then I believe God will ask me, **"Dale, do you have a death to pay for your sins?"** He will ask me this because Romans 6:23 explains, *"The wages of sin is death, but the free gift of God is salvation through Jesus Christ our Lord."* I have sins, and need a death to pay for my sins. Jesus was the sinless Son of God. *"He was tempted in all things even as we are, but was without sin"* (Hebrews 4:15). So I have sins but no death. And Jesus has a death, but no sins. Jesus has made me an offer I can't refuse. He will pay for my sins by letting me trust in His death to pay my sin debt. So I will tell God, "I have a death to pay for my sins. The death of Your sinless only and beloved Son, Jesus." Then I will quote the most important verse in the Bible and totally give my eternal fate over to God with thanksgiving. *"For God so loved the world that He gave His only begotten Son that whosoever believes in Him might not perish, but have everlasting life"* (John 3:16).

IDENTITY

Identity? What does it mean?
I once was sin stained. Now I'm clean.

Identity? How am I now?
There are some things I can't allow.

Identity? What can I do?
I can believe in God and you.

Identity? What lies ahead?
It means I'll never be caught dead.

Identity? What of today?
I follow Christ, my Life, my Way.

Identity? I know my name.
It is "a son of God" the same

The Messiah explained, *"I am the way, the truth and the life. No man comes unto the Father but by Me"* (John 14:6).

Without Christ the way – there is no going. Without Christ the truth – there is no knowing. Without Christ the life, there is no living.

*"But as many as received Him, **to them gave He power to become the sons of God**, even to them that believe in His name"* (John 1:12).

KILL "SOMEONE" WHO CAN'T FIGHT?

Today you contemplate an act
    which can't go in reverse.
You chose to be a living womb
    or cold metallic hearse.

You chose to birth a Soul who needs
    sweet lullabies at night.
Or else you chose to have cruel knives
    kill Someone who can't fight.

You chose to listen to a heartbeat
    crying out for care.
There's Someone growing within you
    who trusts you to be fair.

Your Child needs you more than ever
    as you make your choice
To let your Child live and hug you…
    love you with his voice.

Some say, "Your Child's just a fetus*,
    unformed, just a blob."
Some Hitler like abortionists
    are working for the mob.

The underworld has an interest
    in the future Dead.
It's time to touch your swelling bosoms.
    Will Someone be fed?

Did you know that a doctor who
    delivers Children live
Earns less than half of doctors whose
    small Patients don't survive?

What motivates the couns'lor who wants
    you to kill your Child?
Is she seeking affirmation? Did
    she do something wild?

Search your couns'lor's memories
    and ask if she once had
An abortion? Would she be jealous
    if you were good, not bad?

Would she be hopping, red faced envious
    if you caused her strife
And chose to give your child a chance
    to live a love filled life?

And if she senses that you've panicked
    and you're filled with fear…
Insist that she reflect and tell you
    if she's shed a tear

Of longing for Someone that she once
    carried 'neath her heart.
Ask if she ever felt that Someone's
    missing…that a part

Of her is gone? Ask if she's sure
    that what she did was best.
Ask her about the lonely nights
    when it's so hard to rest.

If Someone didn't kill a Child, then
    who is it that's missed?
What feeling person thinks that death
    is preferred to being kissed?

When women are made victims by
    heartless abortion mills,
They tend to drink a bit too much,
    and take too many pills.

Be sure to ask your couns'ler if she
    knows those who abuse.
If there was not a real death,
    is pregnancy a ruse?

The bottom line is simply this,
    "Just when does life begin?"
How can an egg and sperm unite
    in dishes made of tin…

Then be transplanted to a womb
    and swift become a child
Unless, that Egg that's fertilized
    was living? I'm so riled!

Some advocates who are pro-choice
    suggest it's best to kill!
Leave that abortuary now!
    I pray you'll feel a chill

Right down your spine…Stand straight and tall
    and run! Don't walk away!
Within a few short precious weeks
    there'll be a bright birth day.

*Fetus is Latin for "small Child"

LOVE YOUR AMAZING MOM PROGRAM (LAMP)

Instead of printing money, it is better for America to add more taxpayers. I challenge anyone to come up with a better solution to our fiscal dilemma than this program.

The purpose of this program is to reward mothers for giving birth to their children. In the case of a mother who lets her child be adopted, she, the birth mom will get the annual reward. The program is simple:

1. Each child whose birth mom is still living will register with his or her mom by March 15, in order to qualify to get three percent of the federal income tax that child pays in to the federal government that year. (Suppose a man pays $100,000 in federal income tax on a given year. By Labor Day that year the IRS will postmark a check for $3,000 to his birth mother. It does not matter how many children a mother has who pay federal income tax on a given year. She gets a separate check for three percent of the income tax paid for each child.

There will be no limit on how much a mother might get from any child. The funds sent to the mother will be tax free. (We anticipate that retailers will get a nice bump when the mothers get their checks. If a mother does not yet own a home, we recommend that she banks part of that LAMP check to enable her child or children to help her buy a home.)

2. The program is voluntary. Both the mother and her individual working children who pay federal income tax must register together in order for the mother to get her LAMP CHECK.

3. The advantage of this program to the country is simple. It will motivate mothers to have more children and reward them when they do. It will motivate mothers to encourage their children to do well in school and take special training if needed in order to get higher paying jobs. It will motivate mothers to have their children when they are younger.

4. I envision a voice vote by the members of the senate and house to pass this bi-partisan legislation unanimously.

It will be administered by the Internal Revenue Service. 100% of all federal taxes will be paid to the IRS. But on Labor Day the IRS will send 3% of the federal tax to the mother of each of her income tax paying children. Registration for the program must be completed by March 15. There will be no grace period if the registration is not completed on time. But they can register for the next year.

Let's take our hats off to our AMAZING MOMS!!!

Of all the things which an OB/GYN doctor does during the course of his or her professional life, what do you think is the single most important activity? I would suggest it is helping a mother birth a healthy full term child. But some doctors instead decide they are qualified to decide if a child should be aborted instead of being born. Are they right to make this decision?

"For You, O Lord, are my hope, O Lord, from my youth. Upon You who took me from my mother's womb. My praise is continually of You" (Psalms 71:5-6).

2020, THE TURNAWAY STUDY

By Diana Greene Foster, PhD (ten years, a thousand women and the consequences of having or being denied an abortion.)

I wish to compliment her on collecting a lot of research and statistics on the subject of abortion. She has made a good start. Now I suggest she continue her research and bring her conclusions up to date. I am happy to share my research with her.

"This book is about women who come in just under the clinic's deadline and received a wanted abortion, and what happens to those who arrive at the very same clinics just a few days or weeks in pregnancy and are turned away. It is also a book about the state of abortion access in our country and the people whose lives are affected by it." (p.2)

I wish to compliment Doctor Foster for including the following information in my favorite page in her insightful book, (p.204). She could have omitted it. How long after the abortion was denied did it take for one third of the mothers to stop wanting an abortion? I quote, "One week after being denied an abortion, nearly two-thirds of women report that they still wanted an abortion. BUT SIX MONTHS LATER, WHEN ALL HAD GIVEN BIRTH, JUST ONE IN EIGHT (12%) WISH THEY COULD HAVE HAD THE ABORTION. FIVE YEARS LATER, ONLY ONE IN TWENTY-FIVE (4%) WISH THEY COULD HAVE HAD THE ABORTION...Sue from Missouri expressed a similarly fierce love for her second son whom she conceived within months of delivering her first. It was terrifyingly bad timing for Sue, but ultimately she's 'Relieved that what happened, happened. Just all of the cute quirky things that he does, and how he makes me smile, and the things I would have missed out on...It breaks my heart that I actually thought about having an abortion.'"

In the interests of being thorough I would have asked the women in her survey who have all had abortions the following questions:
• What percentage after five or more years were glad

they had been given the abortion? BASIC PRINCIPLE: HAPPINESS ISN'T HAVING WHAT YOU WANT, IT IS WANTING WHAT YOU HAVE. Just because on the date of their abortion, the mothers wanted the procedure does not mean as they look back over their decision, that they wanted what they had. (My readers will be excited to compare which group was happier, those who were given or those who were denied an abortion.)

- Next ask what percentage of the women were unable to conceive a child.
- What percentage, if any, had to pay for help to conceive a child? Describe and tell what it cost.
- And what percentage were unable to carry one or more future children they conceived to full term? Did any future children have birth defects? If any were born prematurely, describe what happened and the cost.
- BASIC PRINCIPLE: Look at the Howard University study which showed black women over 50 who were given abortions were 4.7 times more likely to have breast cancer than black women who never had one. Dr, Foster's survey focuses on the results within the first five years after a mother has an abortion. As my research shows, the danger of getting breast cancer continues as the mother passes age fifty.
- Regarding the effects of Post Abortion Syndrome (pp.139-142) what are the specific symptoms they have experienced?

This study omitted reporting on the lives of the children whom their mother initially tried to abort. How can a study on the abortion omit interviewing the children whose lives were saved and sharing a few of their photos? If Doctor Foster wishes to rectify this for example, by setting up a web page with photos of some of the children and their comments about whether or not they are pleased to be alive I will donate a thousand dollars to help cover this expense. She does mention that one reason such a low percentage of women who birth their children offer them up for adoption as being that the mothers were pleasantly surprised at how warmly their family members reacted to their babies. Finally, I urge her to be more inclusive and add comments from those who adopted infants whose lives were saved. Surely these parents deserve to share their opinions and tell how long it took them to finally get their child.

I discuss the negative side effects of the abortion pill on p.114 of this book. You may also research these issues on the internet.

Those who suggest having a chemical abortion as a fast, simple, procedure gloss over many points. By looking inside the front cover of my book, CHOOSE LIFE, we learn HOW VARIOUS TYPES OF ABORTION DAMAGE MOTHERS.

CARING CLINICAL COUNSELOR'S FAILURE

The pro-life folks who volunteer to stand by the doors to the abortion facilities are encouraged to dress well, be poised, prayed up and confident. One of the most attractive even-tempered confident counselors who volunteered noticed what appeared to be a mother bringing in her daughter, approaching the entrance. The counselor prepared a friendly, caring greeting. But then was overcome with emotion and started weeping so much that she could not speak as the two walked past her through the door.

She was embarrassed and felt like a failure because she was unable to even say a single word to encourage them to choose life. After sitting in the reception area a few minutes, the mother took her daughter by the hand and said, "We need to go. Now!"

The mother walked up the counselor and said, "When we were walking towards the door, I saw you. I had prepared words to tell you to leave us alone and not bother us. But your tears turned my heart!"

The weeping counselor hugged them both and explained, "I never wept like this during the years that I have come here to talk with people entering the facility. But I just felt so badly about what you might do...I couldn't speak."

The tears of a caring counselor vanquished the heart of those planning to have an abortion. What a counselor is feeling towards those entering such a business trumps any amount of words they can share.

Select an organization from the RESOURCE CENTER. Give them a call. These kind understanding volunteers are waiting to hear your story. You are not alone.

Review what the abortionist offers you. Compare its value to the following: I believe that before I was conceived, the Creator planned that I should write CHOOSE LIFE and that you should be reading it at this precise minute. In the same way, before your unborn child was conceived the Lord planned out amazingly wonderful specific things which your child would do during his or her lifetime. Ecclesiastes 3 says, *"For everything there is a time. A time be born and a time to die...A time to embrace and a time to refrain."* I embrace you with my words. You are not alone. My mom died at age 98 at 6:45 am on Thanksgiving Day 2015. I was holding her hand. May your unborn child be holding your hand or the hand of the mother who adopted her when you or she passes into eternity.

Imagine an abortionist dressed in his scrubs is standing before you. One of his hands is on a cart with the tools of his trade and a plastic tray on which he will place the dismembered remains of your child. He doesn't care if he will rob your child of life or you of your health. He speaks, "I am here to offer you a safe abortion." (He will likely not offer to show you the ultrasound of your child or offer you the privilege of hearing your baby's heartbeat.) His other hand is stretched out towards you anticipating you will give him cash.

Next to the abortionist stands Jesus. He is holding your child out for you to take and love. Your breasts are beautifully enlarged and engorged. You notice Jesus' hands have nail scars and His eyes are filled with expectant tears. Your child is crying and hungry for your sweet warm breast milk. Your child's hand reaches out to touch your face and heart.

CHOOSE ONE!

May God give you the courage to always do the right thing and bless you, your growing family, friends, finances, faith life, health and all you dream and do. "No woman should feel so alone, coerced or so hopeless that she ends her child's life through abortion." (Heartbeat International).

Dale Stone
Choose1Life@outlook.com
Father's Day 2022.
Let's unite to save lives!

Please retake the pre-reading survey on page 3 of this book and email me if your views have changed.

Has reading CHOOSE LIFE changed your views on abortion? If so and you wish to send a sentence or two recommending CHOOSE LIFE to others facing a crisis pregnancy, I would be happy to consider publishing your endorsement in the next edition of CHOOSE LIFE or in my CHOOSE LIFE blog at CHOOSE1LIFETODAY.org. (See also p.194.)